Defy Aging Naturally

A Practical Guide to Creating and Sustaining Health

Michael Tannin

Table of Contents

Introduction

It is never too late to embrace a healthier lifestyle and the potential for a longer, healthier life! Now is the time—regardless of your age—to adopt healthy habits that can enhance graceful aging and reduce signs of illness. Contrary to common belief, adopting this lifestyle does not require excessive medications or difficulty. All you need is accurate information and guidance.

Aging—a natural part of life—can be accompanied by increased strength and vitality, which are achievable. Like any endeavor, success in aging requires starting early. While you cannot avoid getting older, you do not have to "get old," and this remarkable phase should not define you.

As you approach your golden years, taking ownership of your health empowers you to lead a fulfilling life. Driven by a strong desire to help you live your best life, I am offering a practical guide to creating and sustaining healthy living!

Defy Aging Naturally has been written to present not just an overview but a comprehensive insight into healthy aging. Beginning with a solid foundation, the first section introduces healthy aging, covering its importance, dispelling misconceptions, and providing guidance on living life on your own terms.

As you move forward, you will explore the science of aging, exploring biological processes and influencing factors, and gaining a deeper understanding of cellular aging. You will discover Geneticist Bennett's profound insights into the mechanics of aging, appreciating its contemporary perspective on healthy aging.

The impact of positive thinking on healthy aging is profound. You will delve into current research on this topic, along with strategies for cultivating a healthy mindset and overcoming age-related biases and stereotypes. Your brain plays a central role in aging, so you will also explore strategies for maintaining brain health and providing it with the necessary nutrients to function optimally during your golden years. Given the impact of nutrition, I will guide you through the essential nutrients for healthy aging, offering recommended tips for maintaining a nutritious diet as you grow older. This includes a deeper exploration of macro and micronutrients.

Undoubtedly, physical activity is beneficial, but how do you choose the right exercise? The next section introduces you to the benefits and types of exercises recommended for various age groups. If you have tried exercises before but struggled to stick with them, fear not! I have included tips to help you integrate exercise into your daily routine.

Your social connections and emotional well-being are crucial, and you will gain an in-depth understanding about that. You will leave with practical skills for enhancing emotional well-being. As you age, you may face challenges with sleep and rest, but I have got you covered with tips and strategies to improve sleep hygiene and manage sleep disorders.

Finally, this guide will conclude with an overview of chronic diseases associated with aging, strategies for preventing and managing these conditions, and the importance of regular healthcare checkups.

Embark on a rewarding journey with this refreshingly practical and straightforward book. The advice offered here is attainable, leaving you feeling energized and inspired. This guide is your ideal companion that you will want to refer to often!

Now is the time to prioritize your health and honor your body, ensuring you age well and live a healthy life!

Chapter 1:

Introduction to Healthy Aging

Introduction —

Aging is a beautiful process that should not be feared. Many people dread the later stages of life, imagining it solely as a time of physical decline and dependency. This misconception is far from reality. Once you dispel such myths, you can embrace the fulfilling journey of aging.

Healthy aging is a holistic experience. It is not just about avoiding hospital visits; it is about maintaining vitality and well-being. One common myth is that aging inevitably leads to illness and financial strain. However, this is not true. That is why I want to introduce you to the concept of "Healthy Aging."

As you embark on this beautiful journey, it is essential to make choices that nurture both your body and mind. This process empowers you to take control of your life, living with purpose and meaning regardless of age. By now, I am sure you are feeling optimistic about your aging process. Let us delve into the art of aging gracefully.

Definition of Healthy Aging

Healthy aging is a dynamic process aimed at optimizing opportunities to maintain and enhance physical and mental health, independence, and overall quality of life across the lifespan (Pan American Health Organization, n.d.). Healthy aging involves developing and maintaining the functional ability that enables well-being in older age (World Health Organization, 2020).

From the definitions of healthy aging, it is evident that aging can enhance overall health and well-being by ensuring continued fitness and capability as one grows older. Beyond avoiding illness, it encompasses physical, mental, and social aspects of life. As we age, maintaining a connection with the world and independence is crucial; thus, there is a strong incentive to prioritize holistic health.

There is no set age for being "old." It is a label you embrace when you allow it. Consider this scenario: You might meet a 70-year-old man who exudes physical strength, leaving you amazed at his capabilities, while another person of the same age struggles with basic tasks. The difference lies in how they have approached their aging process. Aging well is not tied to reaching a specific age; it is about taking control whenever you choose to start.

Your environment significantly influences how you age. Surrounding yourself with supportive individuals who can contribute to your physical, mental, and emotional well-being is crucial. Now that we understand what healthy aging entails, let us delve deeper into why embracing the process of aging gracefully is essential.

Importance of Healthy Aging

Healthy aging is crucial for maintaining well-being and independence as we grow older. By prioritizing nutrition, exercise, social connections, and stress management, individuals can enhance their quality of life and vitality. Below are some key aspects highlighting the importance of healthy aging.

1. Improves the Quality of Life

One of the greatest benefits of healthy aging is the dramatic improvement in your quality of life. Imagine becoming more independent as you age—it is entirely possible. You will not need assistance to navigate stairs or have doctors advising you to limit activities you love just because of your age. If you enjoy hiking, you can continue for as long as you choose, provided you take control of your aging process.

2. Enhances Physical Health

While it is true that aging increases susceptibility to various diseases, it is not inevitable to develop them. Many people live long lives without experiencing chronic illnesses, and you can achieve the same. The true joy of aging is being able to fulfill dreams and goals, thanks to accumulated experience, knowledge, and financial stability. However, if you find yourself dealing with health issues, it not only affects your physical well-being but also diminishes your peace and happiness.

3. Promotes Mental Stability

Many myths surround aging, including the belief that it inevitably leads to mental decline. However, adopting a healthy aging lifestyle can significantly improve cognitive and mental well-being. Imagine maintaining sharpness and vibrancy as you age—this not only brings personal joy but also garners admiration from others who witness your vitality and clarity of mind.

4. Ensures Financial Stability

Health truly is wealth. Some people depend on medications to survive, much like we rely on food. However, these medications can be costly, and whether financially stable or not, individuals often struggle to afford them. Imagine being older and healthier—this not only reduces the need for expensive medications and caretakers but also decreases the risk of losing employment due to perceived incompetence before retirement age. Embracing a healthier lifestyle can help avoid these challenges altogether.

5. Facilitates Lifelong Dreams

Just because you are getting older does not mean you have to let go of your dreams and aspirations. If you want to travel the world and explore new horizons, you can. Instead of letting age hold you back from the things you love, now is the time to say "no" to limitations and set the foundation for a purposeful and adventurous life in your later years.

Common Misconceptions About Aging

What often scares people about aging are the misconceptions about how it will affect them. While there may be challenges, it is important to focus on the positive aspects of aging. By adopting healthy habits and lifestyle choices, you can enhance your healing, well-being, and overall quality of life as you age. Let us debunk some common myths about aging.

Myth #1: Older People Lose Touch With the World

If you want proof that this statement is false, just search on Google or YouTube for older people creating viral and exciting content online. The truth is, aging does not mean you are confined to your bed or isolated from the world. As you grow older, you have opportunities to engage in outdoor activities like jogging, hiking, or exploring new places. Alternatively, you can choose to stay indoors and enjoy the vast array of experiences and connections available through the Internet.

Myth #2: Older People Prefer Small Circles

If you are someone who values the company of friends and loved ones, it is unlikely that as you grow older, you will prefer solitude over companionship. The joy of aging lies in maintaining strong social connections and enjoying the company of those around you. It is important to stay socially connected with friends and nurture the relationships you have built over time. Having people with whom you can share feelings, have conversations, and enjoy activities brings happiness and fulfillment as you age. With old age, the saying "the more, the merrier" holds true.

Myth #3: With Age, Mental and Physical States Worsen

There is a common stereotype that posture worsens with age, but aging does not always mean becoming feeble or losing vitality. You can prevent slouching as you age by adopting healthy habits such as regular exercise and a balanced diet, which we will explore further in this book. Aging can actually mean continuing activities like hiking or going to the gym. By taking proactive steps, you can enjoy the aging process while continuing to do the things you love.

Myth #4: Older People Develop Alzheimer's and Dementia

While the risk of developing Alzheimer's and dementia increases with age, not everyone will experience these conditions in their lifetime. You can enjoy your later years without forgetting your loved ones or experiencing significant memory loss.

Now that you have a better understanding of these myths, it is time to release any fears and embrace your journey of aging.

Start Living the Story of How You Want Your Life to Be

As you embrace the beauty of aging, cherish each experience as a phase of life. Be intentional about cultivating good health and well-being at every step. Take control of your life to craft a narrative filled with meaning, splendor, and happiness.

In addition to maintaining physical fitness, as you grow older, taking proper steps allows you to nurture your spirit and ensure each moment contributes to a vibrant story of healthy aging.

Now that you grasp the foundational aspects of healthy aging, the next chapter will delve into the mysteries of aging and the science behind it. Get ready to explore the wonders within the body that contribute to this beautiful aging process—so grab some popcorn and join us!

Chapter 2:

The Science of Aging

Consumers spend billions of dollars annually on anti-aging remedies and treatments. Creams, Botox, and hair dyes are the new go-to solutions. Some invest in hair Botox for rejuvenation, others opt for anti-aging creams to minimize fine lines, and many rely on hair dyes to achieve a younger look. While these treatments can effectively create the appearance of youth, none can truly turn back the hands of time. That is the reality.

You may wonder: "If these remedies cannot get to the root, then what is the science behind aging?" Scientists are tirelessly working to fully understand the biological causes of aging, and they have made astounding progress. The results of their research are mind-boggling and offer beautiful insights into the remarkable capabilities of human cells.

In this chapter, you will explore the biological process of aging, the factors influencing it, and why Geneticist Bennett's understanding of cellular aging is so vital. Yes, you are in for a pleasant ride!

Biological Processes of Aging

Irrespective of what you do, your body will undergo several changes. Starting around age 20, lung tissues begin to lose elasticity, lung function diminishes, and muscles around the rib cage start to deteriorate. Additionally, the rapid production of digestive enzymes slows down, affecting how nutrients are absorbed and the types of food the body can digest without difficulty.

As we age, blood vessels also lose flexibility. For those with a sedentary lifestyle and unhealthy diet, this loss of elasticity can lead to the hardening of the arteries. In women approaching menopause, vaginal fluids decrease, while in men, lean muscle mass thins and sperm production reduces.

Biologists use the concept of aging to explain the process of aging. Simply put, aging is the process of growing old. In biology, aging is defined as the process by which a cell ages and stops dividing but does not die. Over time, these old cells accumulate in tissues throughout the body, leading to the visible signs of aging.

Characteristics of Aging

Below are four characteristics of aging:

1. **Gradual Process:** Aging unfolds slowly over time, marking the natural progression of aging within an organism. This gradual decline encompasses various physiological and biochemical changes.

2. **Universal Nature:** Aging is a fundamental biological phenomenon observed across the plant and animal kingdoms. From leaves yellowing and falling off trees to the graying of hair and loss of muscle mass in humans, it manifests universally.

3. **Resulting Deficit:** As aging advances, organisms experience a cumulative deficit in physiological functions and structural integrity. This deficit often leads to decreased efficiency in processes such as metabolism, immune response, and repair mechanisms.

4. **Internal Origin:** The changes associated with aging originate from within the organism itself. They are driven by intrinsic genetic programs and cellular processes that govern aging, including telomere shortening, oxidative stress, and hormonal shifts.

These characteristics highlight aging as a complex biological process integral to the life cycle of organisms, influencing their growth, development, and eventual decline.

Biological Aging Division

Biological aging can be divided into three types:

1. **Primary Aging:** This is the basic, shared, and inevitable set of declines or gains governed by some maturational process.

2. **Secondary Aging:** This is the result of health habits, disease, or environmental influences. Unlike primary aging, this is not shared by all adults.

3. **Tertiary Aging:** This is the rapid decline in the last few years of a person's life before death.

Types of Aging

There are four different types of aging worth exploring. They accurately describe how our body ages on several levels.

1. **Cellular Aging**

   o A cell can replicate nearly 50 times before the genetic material can no longer be copied accurately. This failure in replication is now regarded as cellular aging, where the cell loses its characteristics. The hallmark of cellular aging is the accumulation of senescent cells.

   o The more damage a cell experiences from free radicals and other environmental factors, the more rapidly cellular aging develops.

2. **Hormonal Aging**

o Hormones play a crucial role in aging, especially during childhood, by helping to build muscles and bones and develop female or male characteristics.

o Over time, the output of several hormones depletes, leading to wrinkles, loss of elasticity, and other skin conditions. This also includes the loss of bone density, muscle tone, and sex drive. It is important to note that sex hormone levels are different for males and females.

3. **Accumulative Damage**

o Aging resulting from accumulative damage, also known as wear and tear, is caused by external factors building up over time. Unhealthy foods, UV radiation, exposure to toxins, and pollution are some factors that negatively impact the body.

o Over time, these factors can damage DNA in cells and undermine the body's ability to repair itself, leading to more rapid aging.

4. **Metabolic Aging**

o As you go about your daily activities, the cells in your body regularly turn food into energy, producing byproducts that can be harmful.

o The metabolization process can lead to cell damage. Some experts believe that by slowing down the metabolic process through calorie restriction, they might be able to slow down aging.

Factors That Influence the Aging Process

Apart from the natural aging process, some factors lead to premature aging. This type is called extrinsic aging.

- **Light**

- **Sun Exposure:** This is the leading factor influencing aging. UV (ultraviolet) light and sunlight can age the skin more rapidly than the natural aging process. The result of this type of influence is called photoaging, and this factor accounts for 90% of changes visibly seen on the skin. UV light destroys skin cells and contributes to premature changes. Additionally, sun exposure increases the risk of skin cancer.

- **HEV and Infrared Light:** High-energy visible (HEV) light, also called blue light, and infrared light account for 10% of skin changes. HEV light emanates from electronic devices like smartphones and the sun, while infrared light is invisible but felt as heat. Although they do not pose an increased risk of cancer, they affect the skin and collagen elasticity.

- **Smoking**

  - The toxins present in nicotine alter the cells in the body, breaking down elastic fibers and collagen in the skin. This leads to a sagging, hollow, wrinkled, and gaunt face.

- **Unhealthy Diet**

  - Diets high in refined carbohydrates or sugar can lead to premature aging. Conversely, diets rich in vegetables and fruits can prevent noticeable premature skin changes.

- **Alcohol**

  - Excessive alcohol intake can lead to dehydration and skin damage over time, resulting in signs of premature aging.

- **Poor Sleep Pattern**

  - Low-quality or insufficient sleep can result in premature aging. For example, not getting enough sleep can cause cells to age quicker and faster.

- **Stress**

o When an individual is stressed, their brain pumps cortisol, the stress hormone. This cortisol blocks collagen and hyaluronan synthase, substances that keep the skin looking vibrant and plump, leading to premature aging.

Some Disorders That Lead to Premature Aging

In some rare conditions, certain disorders can lead to premature aging. These include:

- **Werner Syndrome**

  o A rare, inherited disorder marked by rapid aging starting in early adolescence or young adulthood. Signs include graying hair, shorter-than-average height, skin changes, voice changes, thin arms and legs, and unusual facial features.

- **Bloom Syndrome**

  o A rare genetic disorder characterized by short stature, a red rash over the cheeks and nose, mild immune deficiency, and a high susceptibility to infections.

- **Seip Syndrome**

  o A rare genetic disorder marked by the near-complete absence of body fat at birth.

- **Cockayne Syndrome**

  o **Type I:** Evident in early childhood, ultimately leading to death in early adolescence.

  o **Type III:** A milder form that becomes apparent in a person's later life.

- **Rothmund-Thomson Syndrome**

o   An inherited disorder that negatively impacts several parts of the body, including teeth, eyes, bones, skin, and hair. Early signs include a blistering rash on the face in infancy.

- **Mandibuloacral Dysplasia With Type A Lipodystrophy**

    o An autosomal recessive disorder marked by skeletal abnormalities, craniofacial anomalies, growth retardation, and pigmentary skin changes.

- **Hutchinson-Gilford Progeria Syndrome**

    o A progressive genetic disorder that causes children to age rapidly. It occurs randomly and is not inherited. Symptoms, such as hair loss and slow growth, start to appear in early infancy.

Understanding Cellular Aging

Cellular aging is a fundamental aspect of the body's natural lifecycle, where cells inevitably age as we do. This process, elucidated by renowned geneticist Bennett, emphasizes understanding rather than merely slowing down aging. From birth, the mechanism of cellular aging is ingrained in our biology: As cells carry out their functions, they age. The body is designed to manage aging cells by replacing them with new ones.

What triggers cellular aging? Several factors contribute, including oxidative stress from internal and external sources, DNA damage, and a decline in autophagy—the process by which cells remove damaged components. A crucial aspect of cellular aging is cellular aging, where cells cease dividing to protect themselves and surrounding tissues from replication errors. Senescent cells are larger than non-senescent cells and undergo a process lasting about six weeks, crucially involving accurate DNA replication to maintain organ and tissue health.

Understanding these mechanisms is foundational to promoting healthy living as we age, highlighting the intricate interplay of cellular processes in the aging process.

The Three Causes of Cell Aging

Now, let us explore the three causes of cell aging, mentioned above, in more detail:

1. **Oxidative Stress:** Oxidative stress is a primary trigger of cell aging. It occurs when reactive oxygen species (ROS)—molecules produced during normal cell metabolism or from external sources like UV radiation or pollution—overwhelm the cell's antioxidant defenses. ROS can damage DNA, proteins, and lipids, leading to mutations and impairments in cellular function. Cells respond to oxidative stress by halting replication to prevent the propagation of damaged DNA, thereby safeguarding genetic integrity.

2. **DNA Damage:** DNA damage occurs naturally during cellular replication and from exposure to environmental factors like UV light and chemicals. Telomeres—protective caps at the ends of chromosomes—shorten with each cell division. As telomeres shorten, cells receive signals to cease replication, preventing errors in DNA transcription and cellular dysfunction. Without sufficient telomere length, cells can continue dividing uncontrollably, contributing to aging and potentially cancerous growth.

3. **Decline in Autophagy:** Autophagy, or "self-eating," is a cellular process crucial for maintaining cellular health by removing damaged organelles and proteins. As cells age, their ability to perform autophagy declines, leading to the accumulation of dysfunctional components and waste products within the cell. This buildup impairs cellular function, hinders DNA replication, and can trigger cellular aging—where cells enter a state of irreversible growth arrest.

Understanding these causes of cell aging highlights the intricate processes involved in maintaining cellular health and longevity. Addressing oxidative stress, managing DNA damage, and supporting autophagy are crucial strategies in promoting healthy aging at the cellular level.

Addressing the Misconception About Cellular Aging

Cellular aging and apoptosis are two distinct processes that play crucial roles in cellular aging and maintenance. Understanding their differences helps in approaching healthy aging with clarity:

1. **Cellular Aging**

   o **Definition:** Cellular aging refers to the state where a cell stops dividing but remains metabolically active and functional.

   o **Purpose:** Senescent cells cease replication to prevent the propagation of damaged DNA and maintain genetic stability.

   o **Characteristics:** While senescent cells are no longer capable of dividing, they continue to perform their specialized functions in the body. They are not dead cells but are less efficient than younger, replicating cells.

   o **Role in Aging:** Accumulation of senescent cells is associated with aging-related decline in tissue function and contributes to age-related diseases.

2. **Apoptosis**

   o **Definition:** Apoptosis, or programmed cell death, is a controlled process where cells self-destruct in response to specific signals.

   o **Purpose:** Apoptosis occurs to remove damaged, infected, or unnecessary cells without causing harm to neighboring healthy cells.

   o **Characteristics:** Unlike aging, apoptosis is a regulated and orderly process. It helps maintain tissue homeostasis by removing cells that are potentially harmful or no longer needed.

o **Role in Aging:** Apoptosis plays a crucial role in eliminating cells that may become cancerous or dysfunctional due to age-related damage.

In summary, cellular aging and apoptosis are mechanisms that manage cellular health and aging. Aging prevents damaged cells from replicating further, while apoptosis removes cells that pose a risk to tissue integrity. Understanding these processes aids in promoting strategies to support healthy aging and mitigate age-related cellular decline.

Healthy Living and Aging Cells

Aging cells are a natural part of human life, where cells gradually lose their efficiency and are replaced by newer ones. While you cannot stop cells from aging, adopting healthy lifestyle practices can help delay premature aging and support overall cellular wellness.

Here are key points to consider:

- **Avoiding Premature Aging:** Certain behaviors and environmental factors can accelerate cellular aging. These include excessive sun exposure leading to sunburns, smoking, using tanning beds, chronic stress, obesity, and substance abuse. These activities place additional stress on cells, triggering premature aging processes.

- **Embracing Aging:** Instead of fearing aging cells and an aging body, recognize them as a testament to a life well-lived. Aging is a natural process that signifies maturity and experience.

- **Protecting Cellular Health:** This guide emphasizes practical ways to protect and support cells as they age. This includes making lifestyle choices that promote overall health and cellular resilience.

In the upcoming chapter, we will go over practical strategies for healthy aging, starting with cultivating the right mindset. This foundational approach will set the stage for exploring how various lifestyle choices—from nutrition and exercise to stress management—affect cellular health and overall well-being.

Chapter 3:

Mindset for Healthy Aging

Our journey through life evokes a myriad of emotions as we age—from fear and excitement to nostalgia. Yet, hidden within the folds of time lies an undiscovered truth: Aging offers boundless opportunities for wisdom and understanding that only experience can impart.

Healthy aging transcends mere physical wellness; it encompasses cultivating a resilient, optimistic mind that continually seeks growth and accomplishment. Imagine awakening each day without fear of aging but with a steadfast determination to conquer challenges and radiate confidence. Achieving this state is not instantaneous; it requires intentional effort.

This is where the power of mindset comes into play—a potent tool that reframes the relentless passage of time as an inspiring and fulfilling journey. It empowers individuals to view aging not as a decline, but as an opportunity for personal evolution and enrichment. By cultivating a positive mindset, individuals can embrace each day with purpose and optimism, seeing every challenge as a chance for growth and every achievement as a testament to resilience.

The Power of Positive Thinking

A positive mindset is indeed one of the most powerful tools anyone can wield. Consider visionaries like Thomas Edison or Karl Benz: Before inventing world-changing technologies, they did not simply wake up and decide, "Today, I will invent the electric bulb." Their achievements were born from perseverance, dedication, and above all, positive thinking. It is this mindset that empowers us to set ambitious goals and believe in our ability to achieve them.

I encourage you to approach aging with the same energy. Let go of the old mindset that views aging as a dreadful journey toward the great beyond. Nobody remains a child forever; aging is inevitable for everyone. The key is to utilize your time effectively and embrace the opportunities each phase of life brings.

So, how does positive thinking transform your outlook on aging?

Firstly, what is positive thinking? Positive thinking involves seeking solutions optimistically. When faced with challenges, you do not ignore them but actively seek solutions. Taking control of your life and pursuing your dreams requires a positive mindset. It is about believing in yourself and your ability to overcome obstacles.

Have you ever felt a rush of energy coursing through your body after hearing someone speak about the power of positive thinking? If so, let that feeling be your reminder that a positive mindset is crucial for healthy aging. Having a positive outlook means seeing the good in things and people, and fostering hope and faith that things will work out.

Beyond opening up possibilities, a positive mindset is vital for your health and well-being. It can boost self-esteem, enhance physical health, and brighten your overall outlook on life. By cultivating positivity, you can ward off persistent sadness, elevate your mood, and cultivate healthier relationships with friends, family, and coworkers.

As one thinks, so will they be!

Strategies for Cultivating a Healthy Mindset

Engaging in mindfulness practices, challenging negative thought patterns, setting realistic goals, practicing gratitude, surrounding yourself with positive influences, seeking support when needed, and prioritizing self-care are effective strategies for nurturing a healthy mindset.

1. Cut Back on Anything That Robs You Off Your Energy

Developing a positive mindset becomes challenging when constantly stressed. Picture finishing a strenuous activity, chest heaving from exhaustion—hardly the ideal moment to focus on goals. Start by identifying energy-draining factors in your life, whether work, school, activities, or certain individuals.

Some habits, like excessive phone use or reliance on alcohol, subtly harm mental health. Recognize these energy-sapping influences and take proactive steps to cut them out. Replace them with activities like meditation and prioritizing important tasks. You will be amazed at how dramatically your mindset can improve.

2. Be Intentional About Living a Healthy Life

It might sound surprising, but your daily diet, activity level, and other factors significantly influence your mindset. Before focusing on developing your mindset, it is crucial to step back and assess if your lifestyle aligns with healthy living standards. Ask yourself these questions: Am I getting enough sleep? Do I consume fruits and vegetables regularly? Am I staying hydrated? Have I reduced my alcohol intake? How often do I exercise?

Take a critical look at your lifestyle and identify areas that could be affecting you. If, for instance, you currently exercise only once a month but aim to increase it to four times a month, start by gradually improving in those areas. The goal is to avoid adding stress, so make changes that do not overwhelm you. Once you commit to prioritizing your health, you will experience a positive shift in your mindset that will reinforce your new habits.

3. Spend Quality Time With Friends and Family

The time spent with loved ones is truly invaluable. It is during these moments that we feel immense joy and happiness as we share thoughts and emotions with them. Conversely, isolating oneself can profoundly impact mental health. If you find yourself struggling with a negative mindset, consider surrounding yourself with people you care about. This does not always require physical meetings; even regular chats or voice and video calls can make a difference.

It is important to avoid distancing yourself from those who care about you, as this can lead to negative outcomes over time. Cultivating healthy relationships is key to personal growth and well-being. Give this approach a try, and you will likely notice a significant improvement in your outlook.

4. Enjoy The Benefits of Social Media

While social media can sometimes harm your mindset, it can also be a positive influence if used wisely. Surround yourself with uplifting movies, music, or podcasts that boost your mood. Be mindful not to let social media consumption become excessive; moderation is key, as too much can be detrimental.

To start your day joyfully, consider reading a book instead of the newspaper. If you prefer staying updated, opt for your favorite podcast or playlist instead of traditional news broadcasts.

5. Work With a Professional Coach

When the process becomes overwhelming, there is no harm in seeking help from a licensed professional coach. Developing a positive mindset requires dedicated effort and breaking old habits. A coach serves as an unbiased guide, offering understanding and strategies to help you excel.

Overcoming Age-Related Stereotypes and Biases

To overcome stereotypes about aging, you can start by challenging the biases ingrained in your mind and embracing the richness that aging offers.

1. Look at the Capabilities of the Person

Often, we tend to judge people's capabilities based on their age. You might assume a man in his early thirties can lift weights better than a man in his late fifties. However, the truth is that the fifty-year-old man could potentially lift weights better than the younger man. It all depends on their individual capabilities and how they have invested in themselves. So, let us eliminate biases based on age when assessing people's abilities.

2. Build More Relationships With People Younger and Older Than You

Often, we naturally gravitate toward peers in our own age group—a tendency that can lead to prejudice based on age differences. It is common to assume that younger individuals may not be interested in connecting with us due to these gaps. However, a simple solution lies in initiating conversations with them first, revealing the richness and wisdom of life experiences that we have to offer. These experiences can greatly enrich their perspectives and foster meaningful connections.

Conversely, forming relationships with older individuals also benefits the younger generation by providing mentors to look up to. Having a guiding figure can be incredibly rewarding and helps younger individuals navigate challenges and gain valuable insights.

3. Get Rid of Negative Stereotypes

Take a moment to identify all your concerns and biases about aging. List them out and address each one individually, aiming to cultivate a positive mindset. For example, if you worry about developing wrinkles as you age, start by gathering information from credible sources or speaking with older individuals to understand the reality. While aging can naturally lead to changes like wrinkles, there are effective ways to mitigate them, such as using quality skincare products and adopting good skin care habits.

4. Be Careful of Your Language

Sometimes, the language we use can inadvertently perpetuate age-related discrimination. Are you frequently using phrases like "When I was much younger" or "While I was still more capable"? Reframing these expressions with a positive mindset can make a difference. Instead of implying that life was better when younger, try saying "While I was in my thirties" or "During my earlier years." This subtle shift can help promote a more inclusive and respectful dialogue about age.

5. Take Pride in Aging

Getting older is not something to be ashamed of. Instead, it should be embraced as a time to gain wisdom and life experience. If you find yourself discriminating against people of a certain age, remember that you too will reach that age eventually. It is important to cultivate a positive mindset now so that you can navigate your life with grace and positivity when you do reach that stage.

To summarize, fostering a positive mindset is crucial for healthy aging. Keep your passion alive, stay open-minded, and find joy in even the smallest things to stay youthful at heart. By nurturing your mental and emotional well-being, you can lead a more purposeful life as you age.

It is important to note that the mindset I have emphasized is closely tied to brain health. In the next chapter, we will explore how to effectively support brain health, ensuring it performs at its peak throughout the day.

Chapter 4:

Maintaining Brain Health

Imagine your brain as the control center of a spaceship, coordinating every thought, memory, movement, and emotion with precision and efficiency. Like any vital system, it requires consistent care and attention to function at its best.

In this chapter, we embark on a journey to explore practical and powerful methods for maintaining and enhancing brain health. We delve deep into various aspects, from effective stress reduction techniques to optimizing nutrition for providing essential brain fuel. We will uncover strategies to sharpen mental focus, combat inflammation that affects brain function, and stimulate the growth of neurons to support cognitive vitality.

Whether your goal is to boost cognitive performance for academic or professional achievements or to ensure your brain remains sharp and agile as you age gracefully, you will find invaluable tips and strategies here.

So, fasten your seatbelt and prepare to empower your brain! Together, we will navigate through evidence-based approaches and practical advice that will help you optimize your brain's health and functionality. Let us unlock the secrets to maintaining a sharp mind and nurturing your brain's potential for years to come.

Importance of Brain Health

As we age, our brain loses elasticity, making it harder to form cognitive connections, maintain focus, and remember. However, prioritizing brain health can significantly delay this cognitive decline. Mental health is just as crucial as physical health—neglecting it weakens the brain, similar to how inactivity weakens muscles.

For older adults, preserving brain health means more than avoiding conditions like dementia; it enhances quality of life. Sharp mental faculties support independence, sound decision-making, and the ability to enjoy daily activities and hobbies.

Furthermore, brain health is closely linked to physical health, promoting better coordination, balance, and emotional well-being, which reduces risks like falls. Activities that challenge the brain—such as puzzles, learning new skills, or socializing—forge new neural connections and bolster cognitive strength.

Prioritizing brain health empowers older adults to sustain mental agility, vitality, and longevity. Let us explore effective strategies for maintaining optimal brain health.

Stress and the Brain

We all experience disorganization and forgetfulness under stress—it is a common response. However, chronic stress can have lasting effects on our brains and memories.

Research has demonstrated that stress alters brain function in both animals and humans. When exposed to life stress or stress induced in research settings (like counting numbers backward), changes in cognition, memory, and attention have been observed (*Protect Your Brain From Stress*, 2018).

Stress not only affects cognition and memory but also increases the risk of anxiety and promotes inflammation, which can contribute to brain and heart conditions over time.

To understand how stress impacts the brain, it is essential to consider its operational mechanism. The human brain functions as a network of specialized units, each responsible for specific tasks. When one part, like the amygdala (responsible for survival instincts), becomes highly active—

such as during perceived danger—it monopolizes energy resources. This leaves other parts of the brain, crucial for memory and cognitive tasks, with insufficient energy to function effectively. Essentially, the brain prioritizes survival over memory formation, leading to forgetfulness and impaired cognitive performance during stressful or traumatic experiences.

How to Protect Your Brain From Getting Damaged by Stress

The best way to manage stress is to minimize factors that exacerbate it. Here are some effective tips to help you manage stress and prevent its harmful effects on your brain:

- **Take Control:** Feeling powerless can amplify stress. Empower yourself by actively seeking solutions to your challenges. Taking action reduces stress levels and restores a sense of control.

- **Get Active:** Physical exercise will not eliminate stress, but it can clear your mind, reduce emotional intensity, and help you approach problems calmly.

- **Prioritize Sleep:** Chronic stress often leads to sleep difficulties, which can worsen stress levels further. Aim for 8 hours of sleep each night, establish a bedtime routine, create a relaxing sleep environment, and avoid caffeine in the evening.

- **Build a Support System:** Connecting with family, friends, and colleagues can provide emotional support and offer new perspectives on your challenges. Talking about your problems with others can lead to solutions while spending time doing enjoyable activities with loved ones can help you unwind and relieve stress.

- **Practice Self-Care:** Balancing work with activities you enjoy is essential for maintaining mental well-being. Make time to relax, socialize, and engage in hobbies. Schedule regular "me time" to recharge and focus on self-care.

Power the Brain With What It Needs

To maintain optimal cognitive function and overall well-being, it is crucial to provide your brain with the nutrients it needs to perform at its peak. Here are key strategies to nourish your brain:

- **Nutrient-Rich Foods:** Imagine your brain as a high-performance engine that requires the right fuel. Focus on a diet rich in nutrients beneficial for brain health:

  o **Omega-3 Fatty Acids:** Found in seafood like tuna, salmon, and flaxseeds, these fats combat age-related cognitive decline and support brain cell function.

  o **Antioxidants:** Berries, leafy greens, and vegetables are rich in antioxidants that protect against oxidative stress and inflammation, which can affect cognitive function.

  o **Vitamins and Minerals:** Ensure your diet includes sources of vitamin B12, vitamin D, and folate, as deficiencies in these nutrients are linked to cognitive impairment.

- **Hydration:** Proper hydration is crucial for brain function. Older adults are more prone to dehydration, which can impact cognitive abilities. Keep a water bottle handy and consider adding flavor with lemon or cucumber to encourage regular hydration.

- **Balanced Meals:** Opt for balanced meals that provide steady energy throughout the day:

  o **Whole Grains:** Foods like oats and quinoa offer a slow release of energy, promoting alertness and focus.

  o **Lean Proteins:** Chicken, fish, and beans are excellent sources of lean protein, essential for repairing and building brain cells.

- o **Healthy Fats:** Nuts, seeds, and olive oil provide essential fats that support brain function and overall health.

- **Supplements:** In some cases, supplements such as omega-3 fish oil or vitamin D may be necessary to fill nutritional gaps. Consult your doctor to determine if supplements are suitable for your individual needs and health status.

By incorporating these strategies into your daily routine, you can support brain health and maintain mental clarity as you age.

Fuel Your Mitochondria Brain Cells

Mitochondria are essential tiny structures found within your cells, comprising up to 10% of your body weight and playing a crucial role in brain function and mental health. Known as the "powerhouse of the cell," mitochondria convert the food you eat into Adenosine Triphosphate (ATP), the primary cellular fuel that powers daily activities. Adequate ATP production is vital for proper brain function, and dysfunction of mitochondria can lead to increased oxidative stress, commonly associated with brain and mental illnesses.

To enhance brain and mental health, consider these lifestyle changes aimed at boosting mitochondrial function:

- **Avoid Poor Quality Foods:** In addition to consuming nutrient-rich whole foods, steer clear of refined sugars, processed foods, trans fats, and oils. These foods can impair mitochondrial efficiency and energy production. Some experts also recommend limiting dairy, gluten, and soy for optimal mitochondrial health (Fallis, 2024).

- **Exercise Regularly:** Regular physical activity boosts oxygen and blood flow to mitochondria, activating pathways that promote mitochondrial biogenesis—the process of creating new mitochondria. Exercise also helps combat age-related muscle decline.

- **Reduce Calorie Intake:** Calorie restriction can enhance longevity by activating stress signals that strengthen mitochondria, prevent damage, and remove dysfunctional ones.

- **Increase Magnesium Intake:** Magnesium, stored primarily in mitochondria, plays a critical role in protecting these cellular powerhouses and enhancing ATP production and transfer. Studies suggest that magnesium deficiency is linked to fewer mitochondria and overall poorer health (George & Heaton, 1975). Incorporate magnesium-rich foods like bananas, avocados, and dark chocolate into your diet.

By adopting these strategies, you can support mitochondrial health, optimize ATP production, and promote overall brain and mental well-being.

Reverse Inflammation for Better Brain Performance

Inflammation is the body's natural defense response to toxins, viruses, bacteria, and other threats. When it occurs in the brain, this process is crucial for protecting brain tissue, managed by its immune system through mechanisms like the blood-brain barrier (BBB), astrocytes, and microglia. However, chronic inflammation can lead to detrimental effects on brain health, including headaches, irritability, brain fog, and reduced focus.

To combat inflammation and support optimal brain performance, consider these tips:

- **Eat Anti-Inflammatory Foods:** Incorporate plenty of fresh vegetables, oily fish (like salmon and mackerel), avocados, berries (especially blueberries), chia seeds, grapes, nuts, coffee, and tea into your diet. These foods are rich in antioxidants and nutrients that help reduce inflammation.

- **Avoid Inflammatory Foods:** Adopting an anti-inflammatory diet involves not only consuming more beneficial foods but also cutting back on inflammatory ones. Reduce your intake of red meat, fried foods, trans fats, and processed foods, which can exacerbate inflammation.

- **Manage Blood Sugar Levels:** Control your consumption of carbohydrates such as white rice, white bread, refined sugar, pasta, and other high glycemic foods. Opt for lean meats, whole grains, and vegetables, which help stabilize blood sugar levels and reduce inflammation.

- **Reduce Stress:** Stress triggers inflammatory responses in the body, including the brain. Practice stress-reducing techniques such as mindfulness, meditation, yoga, and deep breathing exercises to manage stress effectively and mitigate its inflammatory effects.

- **Consider Supplements:** Consult with your healthcare provider about supplements that may help reduce brain inflammation and support cognitive function. Omega-3 fatty acids, curcumin (from turmeric), and resveratrol are examples of supplements known for their anti-inflammatory properties.

By implementing these strategies, you can help reduce inflammation in the brain, enhance cognitive function, and promote overall brain health.

Activities That Promote Neuron Growth

One of the most fascinating aspects of our brains is their ability to continually form new neuronal connections, a phenomenon known as neuroplasticity. This remarkable capability allows us to enhance cognitive functions such as processing speed, memory retention, and learning abilities throughout our lives.

To actively promote neuron growth and strengthen existing connections, consider these strategies:

- **Learning New Skills:** Engaging in activities that challenge your brain, such as learning a musical instrument, mastering a new language, or exploring creative hobbies like painting, stimulates the growth of new neurons and reinforces neural pathways.

- **Aerobic Exercise:** Regular aerobic exercise not only improves cardiovascular health but also boosts neuroplasticity. It enhances blood circulation to the brain and triggers the release of growth factors that support neuron production. Studies have shown that aerobic exercise increases neuronal production in brain regions like the hippocampus, which is crucial for memory and learning (Yau et al., 2014).

- **Meditation:** Chronic stress can impair neurogenesis in brain regions like the hippocampus. Meditation practices have been found to increase gray matter volume and hippocampal size, likely due to their stress-reducing effects (Luders et al., 2009). By promoting relaxation and mental clarity, meditation supports brain health and plasticity.

- **Social Interaction:** Maintaining social connections and engaging in meaningful conversations stimulate brain activity and promote neuroplasticity. Social engagement encourages the brain to adapt to new information and challenges, thereby enhancing cognitive abilities.

Just as a spaceship's control center requires meticulous care to function optimally, your brain thrives when given the right attention and resources. Practicing mindfulness to manage stress, providing your brain with nutritious foods, and fostering flexibility through learning and socializing are practical ways to enhance its performance and resilience over time.

In the next chapter, we will delve into the pivotal role that a healthy diet plays in defying the aging process and preserving cognitive vitality as we grow older.

Chapter 5:

Holistic Nutrition

Eating a nutritious, balanced diet is crucial for staying healthy as you age. During this phase of life, your appetite, feeding habits, and nutritional needs change in several ways. Emphasizing the preparation of balanced, nutritious meals that fulfill dietary desires is essential for older adults.

This chapter explores the importance of nutritious diets, key nutrients for healthy aging, and tips for maintaining a balanced feeding plan as you age. From lowering the risk of potential health diseases associated with aging to maintaining a healthy weight and staying energized, you will discover how to support your body through dietary choices.

Importance of a Balanced Diet and Nutrition

Good nutrition is regarded as a fundamental requirement for effective senior care. Research conducted by the National Resource Center on Nutrition, Physical Activity, and Aging shows that one in four elderly Americans has poor nutrition (Gidus, 2019). A study conducted by the University of Bergen in Norway revealed that by adhering to the nutritional guidelines of the Eatwell Guide, a 40-year-old individual could potentially increase their life expectancy by 8.9 years for men and 8.6 years for women of the same age (Flynn, 2023).

Malnutrition, on the other hand, increases the risk of becoming underweight or overweight, weakens muscles and bones, and makes one more vulnerable to diseases. As you age, your metabolism slows down, and your body's ability to absorb nutrients from food decreases. Therefore, older adults must eat nutrient-dense foods to meet the body's daily demands. Additionally, having a balanced meal plan tailored to your unique health needs can help your body adjust and compensate for the reduced functioning of most organs and tissues.

Moreover, as mentioned earlier, growing older predisposes one to a higher risk of malnutrition due to factors such as difficulty chewing and swallowing, limited access to healthy food, and reduced appetite. Access to dietary support and proper nutrition education is essential to maintain a healthy lifestyle.

A healthy diet is also crucial for maintaining cognitive functions in older adults, as it helps improve memory and prevents fatigue. Therefore, it is important to plan meals for seniors, particularly those at risk of developing dementia or already living with it. Cognitive decline, memory problems, and dementia are often associated with malnutrition in older people, highlighting the need for healthy and balanced nutrition.

Critical Nutrients for Healthy Aging

What should your diet look like as you age? To meet your nutritional needs, it is important to limit foods high in processed sugar, salt, and saturated and trans fats. Instead, focus on meals rich in the following crucial nutrients:

Calories	As you age, reduced activity means you need fewer calories to maintain a healthy weight. Consuming more calories than you burn leads to weight gain. Muscle tightness and joint stiffness are common issues that reduce physical activity, leading to fewer calories burned. Senile atrophy (loss of muscle mass due to age) can also lower caloric demand due to slower metabolism.
	However, your body still needs enough energy in the form of calories for basic physiological functions like breathing, walking, and engaging in favorite activities like gardening, playing bingo, or visiting family and friends. Meals that can provide sufficient energy for these activities include pasta, cereals, whole-grain bread, meats, eggs, dairy products, and healthy fats from avocados, nuts, and seed oils.

Protein	Protein is essential for maintaining strong muscles and reducing fatigue symptoms. To keep your muscles active and lessen the risk of falls and injuries, rely on lean or low-fat meats such as grilled chicken, low-fat pork, and salmon. Other good sources include poultry, seafood, eggs, and dairy products like milk, cheese, and yogurt.
Fats	Healthy fats, in moderate amounts, provide energy, especially for seniors with lower calorie intake. They also offer insulation against cold and help absorb certain micronutrients. Abundant sources of healthy fats include tuna, salmon, mackerel, seeds, nuts, avocado, olive oil, and peanut butter. Additionally, fats can be found in sauces, butter, food dressings, milk, and yogurt.
Fibers	Fiber is an essential nutrient that aids in digestion throughout our lives, and it is even more important as we grow older. A lack of fiber in the diet increases the risk of constipation, which can have severe consequences for older adults. There are two kinds of fibers: soluble and insoluble. Soluble fibers help ease bowel movements, while insoluble fibers are the undigested parts of vegetables and fruits that sweep through your intestines. Good sources of fiber include apples, oranges, bananas, leafy vegetables, carrots, celery, pumpkin, potatoes, whole grain bread, cereals, and pasta.
Fluids	Older adults are more likely to have a reduced sense of thirst and a diminished ability to conserve water, which can result in dehydration. Dehydration is a prevalent issue among older adults and can lead to various complications such as delirium, kidney stones, and urinary tract infections. It is essential to drink enough fluids throughout the day, especially during hot weather or when you are sick. Water is the best source of hydration, but you can also meet your fluid needs through soups, fruits, vegetables, teas, milk, juice, and lemonade. Aim for eight glasses of water daily.

Grains	The consumption rate of white flour has grown over time, raising nutritional concerns due to its low nutritional value, which results from removing essential nutrients during bleaching. As a senior, it is important to focus on consuming wholegrain bread, oats, and brown rice for a rich source of carbohydrates.
Calcium	Aging can reduce calcium uptake from food and increase resistance to calcium deposition in the bones. Calcium is crucial for strengthening bones and preventing them from becoming thin, fragile, and brittle. Foods rich in calcium include fortified milk, yogurt, cheese, leafy vegetables, custards, and fish bones.
Magnesium	Magnesium is a vital nutrient essential for muscle and nerve function, playing a crucial role in alleviating soreness, cramps, and muscle tightness. It enhances flexibility and helps prevent tissue injury, which is particularly beneficial for older individuals. Foods rich in magnesium include cashews, whole grains, lentils, soybeans, peanut butter, almonds, and seeds.
Vitamin D	Vitamin D aids in calcium absorption into the bones, promoting bone strength. Most of this nutrient is synthesized by the skin through exposure to the sun's ultraviolet rays. About 80% of the body's vitamin D needs can be met with 10 to 15 minutes of sunlight exposure. Foods like liver, fatty fish, eggs, and vitamin D-fortified foods provide the remaining 20% of vitamin D intake.
Vitamin B	Vitamin B plays a crucial role in maintaining overall health and well-being, particularly as we age. Two key B vitamins, B6 and B12, are essential for brain function, immune system health, and red blood cell production, highlighting the importance of incorporating these nutrients into our diets. • **Vitamin B6:** Important for brain function and immune system health, vitamin B6 helps mitigate

	cognitive decline associated with aging. Sources include fish, potatoes, chickpeas, bananas, and fortified cereals. • **Vitamin B12:** Essential for red blood cell production, vitamin B12 absorption may decrease with age due to reduced gastric acid effectiveness. Foods rich in B12 include fish, beef, poultry, eggs, and dairy products. Vegetarians may consider B12 supplements.
Vitamin K	Vitamin K oversees the synthesis of proteins crucial for tissue repair, blood clotting, and bone health. As people age, decreased physical activity may confine them to a chair or bed, leading to muscle atrophy and reduced strength, which increases the risk of falls and potential injuries. Adequate vitamin K intake supports the synthesis of blood clotting factors essential for wound healing. Another vital role of vitamin K is in preventing bone tissue loss associated with aging. It activates key substances in the body that facilitate calcium uptake into bones and teeth. Foods rich in vitamin K include green leafy vegetables, Brussels sprouts, broccoli, and soybeans.

Tips for Maintaining a Healthy Diet as You Age

As nutritional needs vary with age, strategies for maintaining a well-balanced, healthy diet plan include:

- **Focus on Nutrient-Rich Foods:** As you age, reduce calorie intake while ensuring adequate intake of carbohydrates, proteins, vitamins, minerals, and fats by prioritizing nutrient-dense foods.

- **Increase Fiber Intake:** Fiber is essential for digestive health and managing cholesterol levels.

- **Choose Healthier Convenience Foods:** Opt for nutritious and easy-to-prepare options such as low-sodium canned foods and vegetables, bagged salads, oatmeal, and unsweetened fruits.

- **Stay Hydrated:** Older adults may lose their sense of thirst, leading to dehydration. Drink at least eight 8-ounce glasses of water daily.

- **Consider Supplementation:** Aging can limit nutrient absorption, making supplementation for calcium, magnesium, vitamin D, and vitamin B necessary for those unable to obtain sufficient amounts through diet alone.

Proper nutrition is crucial for maintaining and improving the health of older adults, preventing malnutrition and dehydration, and managing chronic diseases effectively while preserving cognitive function. The next chapter will discuss the macro and micro nutrients essential for daily health and will examine the precise balance of nutrients vital for overall well-being.

Chapter 6:

Macro and Micronutrients That

Promote Daily Health

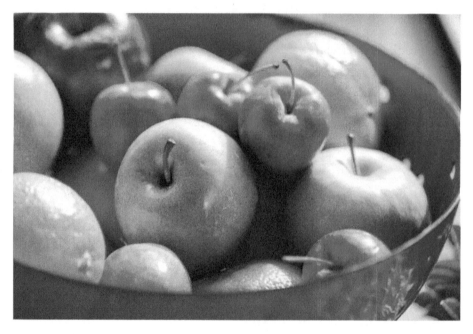

Often, the outcomes we experience in life are a culmination of daily habits and significant decisions made over time. Consistently adopting certain routines can lead to predictable outcomes. When it comes to maintaining optimal health as we age, it becomes crucial to establish a healthy lifestyle early on. This involves engaging in appropriate physical and mental exercises, as well as consuming foods that support daily health.

Committing to a healthy diet as you age goes beyond theoretical knowledge about aging or having the right mindset toward healthy living. While these are foundational aspects, the true essence lies in practical lifestyle practices—the foods you choose to eat, the way you structure your daily life, and the habits you maintain to ensure your body functions at its best.

By prioritizing nutritious foods that provide essential vitamins, minerals, and antioxidants, you can support your body's natural functions and maintain vitality. Incorporating whole grains, lean proteins, colorful fruits and vegetables, and healthy fats into your diet can provide a wide range of nutrients that support overall health and well-being.

Natural Supplements That Benefit Your Body

Natural supplements offer a reliable option for enhancing health by filling nutrient gaps in your diet and potentially providing specific benefits. However, approaching them with a balanced perspective is crucial for ensuring the best outcomes.

Derived from natural sources such as herbs, plants, and minerals, natural supplements typically include vitamins, antioxidants, and other bioactive compounds. They actively support various aspects of health, including immune function, cognitive health, energy levels, and overall well-being.

Compared to pharmaceuticals, natural supplements generally have fewer side effects, though individual responses may vary.

Potential Benefits of Natural Supplement

Natural supplements have gained popularity for their potential health benefits, offering individuals a natural alternative to traditional medication. Below are some benefits of natural supplements:

- **Nutrient Gaps:** Modern diets often lack essential vitamins and minerals. Supplements can effectively bridge these gaps, particularly for individuals with dietary restrictions or limitations.

- **Specific Support:** Certain natural supplements may provide specialized benefits tailored to address specific health concerns.

Understanding the potential benefits and limitations of natural supplements empowers you to make informed decisions about incorporating them into your wellness plan.

Furthermore, the uniqueness of the human body lies in the chain of nutritional and digestive activities that collectively work toward a common goal—the well-being of the mind and body. Every nutrient that enters your body plays an active role in fulfilling the body's dietary requirements for optimal health.

Although nutrients collectively contribute to overall well-being, each plays a distinct role based on its nutritional value and the body's specific needs. Scientific studies and evaluations have classified these nutrients primarily into macro and micronutrients.

Macronutrients

This class of nutrients is required in larger quantities because they primarily provide energy for the body. Energy, biologically known as ATP, is essential for virtually all biological processes and is widely distributed throughout the body. Foods that belong to this group are significant sources of energy. Examples of macronutrients include:

Carbohydrates

Carbohydrates (carbs) often face misconceptions, but they are actually crucial for a healthy diet, playing essential roles in our body's functioning:

Core Functions of Carbohydrates

- **Main Energy Source:** Carbs are broken down into glucose (blood sugar) during digestion. This glucose acts as the primary fuel for your brain, muscles, and central nervous system. It provides 4 kilocalories per gram, which is vital for metabolizing organs such as the brain and kidneys. Excess glucose is stored as glycogen in muscles and the liver for later energy needs.

- **Fiber Powerhouse:** Not all carbs are the same. Complex carbohydrates found in whole grains, fruits, and vegetables are rich in fiber. Fiber promotes gut health, supports digestion, and contributes to feeling full longer, aiding in healthy weight management.

Rich Food Sources

Rich food sources of carbohydrates include oatmeal, bananas, sweet potatoes, quinoa, brown rice, whole grain bread, corn, kidney beans, oranges, and apples.

In summary, carbohydrates are essential for energy provision, digestive health, and overall well-being. Opting for whole, fiber-rich sources and balancing carbohydrate intake with other nutrients is key to maximizing their benefits within a healthy diet.

Fats

Fats are essential macronutrients critical for maintaining overall health and supporting various bodily functions. Composed of carbon, hydrogen, and oxygen atoms, fats are categorized into different types based on their chemical structure and health effects, including saturated, monounsaturated, polyunsaturated, and trans fats, each contributing to overall health.

Core Functions of Fats

- **Energy Storage:** Fats are the most concentrated energy source, providing more than twice the energy of carbohydrates or proteins per gram. They are stored in adipose tissue as triglycerides, serving as a reserve energy source.

- **Vitamin Absorption:** Certain fat-soluble vitamins (A, D, E, and K) require dietary fats for absorption and transport throughout the body.

- **Hormone Production:** Fats act as precursors to hormones and play a crucial role in regulating various bodily functions, including reproduction and metabolism.

Rich Food Sources

Rich food sources of fats include avocado, olive oil, nuts (such as almonds and walnuts), seeds (chia and flaxseeds rich in Omega-3 fats and fiber), fatty fish like salmon, coconut oil, dark chocolate, cheese, and whole eggs. These foods are excellent additions to a balanced diet, providing essential macronutrients necessary for overall health and sustained energy.

In summary, fats are indispensable macronutrients essential for maintaining overall health and supporting vital bodily functions, categorized by their chemical structure and diverse health effects.

Protein

Protein is a crucial nutrient that provides calories for energy and supports overall bodily functions. Often referred to as the building blocks of life, protein plays a fundamental role beyond muscle building, impacting nearly every tissue in the body.

The recommended daily protein intake varies based on factors such as age, activity level, and overall health. A general guideline suggests 0.8 grams of protein per kilogram of body weight per day. For example, a 70 kg (154 lb) person would aim for approximately 56 grams of protein daily. Athletes and individuals with specific health conditions may require higher protein intake, and personalized needs should be determined in consultation with a doctor or registered dietitian.

Core Functions of Protein

- **Muscle Structure and Function:** Proteins are essential for developing, repairing, and maintaining skeletal muscles. They provide the structural framework for muscle tissues and facilitate muscle contraction.

- **Enzymes:** Many enzymes are proteins that catalyze biochemical reactions in the body, aiding in digestion, metabolism, and cellular function.

- **Hormones:** Proteins act as messengers in the form of hormones, regulating various physiological functions such as growth, metabolism, and reproduction.

- **Immune Function:** Antibodies, which are proteins produced by the immune system, help defend the body against harmful pathogens and infections.

Rich Food Sources

Rich food sources of protein include chicken breast, salmon, eggs, Greek yogurt, tofu, lean beef, cottage cheese, lentils, chickpeas, and turkey breast.

Including a variety of protein sources in your diet, balancing intake with other macronutrients, and meeting individual nutritional needs contribute to overall health and well-being.

Magnesium

Magnesium is a crucial macro-mineral required by the body in significant quantities, typically exceeding 400 milligrams daily. It is a fundamental mineral that often takes a backseat to more attention-grabbing nutrients, yet it plays a vital role in over 300 biochemical reactions in the human body. Symbolized as Mg with atomic number 12, magnesium is integral to functions ranging from energy production to nerve function and muscle contraction.

Magnesium deficiency can lead to widespread consequences, but ensuring adequate intake offers numerous health benefits. By incorporating magnesium-rich foods and possibly considering supplements with professional guidance, you can support your body in functioning optimally. Magnesium contributes to essential functions such as regulating blood sugar, maintaining strong bones, and promoting a healthy heart, thereby crucially supporting overall well-being (Ware, 2020).

Core Functions of Magnesium

- **Energy Production:** Magnesium acts as a cofactor in the production of adenosine triphosphate (ATP), which is the primary energy currency of cells. It helps convert carbohydrates, fats, and proteins into energy that the body can use for various functions.

- **Muscle Function:** Magnesium is essential for muscle contraction and relaxation. It regulates the movement of calcium ions in and out of muscle cells, which is critical for proper muscle function. This regulation helps prevent issues like muscle cramps and spasms.

- **Nervous System Support:** Magnesium plays a role in nerve transmission and neuromuscular conduction. It contributes to normal nerve function and helps maintain a calm nervous system, supporting overall neurological health.

- **Bone Health:** Magnesium is involved in bone formation and mineralization. It works alongside calcium and vitamin D to maintain bone density and strength, crucial for skeletal health throughout life.

In summary, magnesium's involvement in these processes underscores its importance in maintaining overall well-being. Ensuring an adequate intake of magnesium-rich foods and, when necessary, considering supplements under professional guidance can support these functions and promote optimal health.

Micronutrients

Micronutrients encompass vitamins and minerals, essential for numerous bodily functions, similar in importance to macronutrients. Dietary guidelines specify varying nutrient requirements based on age and gender.

Inadequate intake of specific micronutrients can lead to malnutrition and associated health issues. While consumed in smaller quantities compared to macronutrients, these vitamins and minerals play equally critical roles in maintaining overall health. Below are a few examples of micronutrients:

Iron

Iron is a micronutrient crucial for both structural and functional roles across all organisms. It plays a pivotal part in oxygen transport and is integral to the composition of oxygen-carrying molecules such as hemoglobin and myoglobin, as well as heme-containing enzymes and non-heme proteins. While required in smaller quantities compared to macronutrients, iron is essential for various physiological processes in plants and animals alike. Foods rich in iron include liver, red meat, and soybean flour.

Core Functions of Iron

- **Production of Hemoglobin:** Iron is essential for the synthesis of hemoglobin, a protein in red blood cells that transports oxygen from the lungs to tissues throughout the body.

- **Production of Myoglobin:** Myoglobin, another iron-containing protein, facilitates oxygen storage and release within muscle cells, supporting muscular function and endurance.

Zinc

Zinc is a chemical element with the symbol Zn and atomic number 30. This micronutrient plays a crucial role in numerous biochemical processes, including amino acid metabolism and gene expression. Foods rich in zinc include oysters, crab, lobster, and other seafood.

Core Functions of Zinc

- **Amino Acid Metabolism:** Zinc aids in the breakdown of amino acids, which are essential for the synthesis of proteins, enzymes, hormones, and other vital molecules.

- **Gene Expression:** Zinc is involved in the regulation of gene expression, which determines how genetic information is translated into functional proteins.

Calcium

Calcium is a mineral with the symbol Ca and atomic number 20. It is classified as a micronutrient and naturally occurs as an alkaline earth metal. Adequate absorption of calcium requires the presence of vitamin D. Foods rich in calcium include cheese, milk, and various dairy products.

Core Functions of Calcium

- **Muscle and Nerve Function:** Calcium is essential for muscle contraction and relaxation, as well as for nerve impulse transmission throughout the body.

- **Blood Circulation:** Calcium supports the movement of blood through the blood vessels, contributing to overall cardiovascular health.

Methylation

According to Miller (2021), methylation is a biochemical process where a group of atoms, including one carbon atom and three hydrogen atoms (CH3), is transferred. This process can alter how molecules function within the body.

Foods rich in methylation-promoting nutrients are crucial for overall well-being and support this biochemical process:

Methylation-Increasing Foods

- **Folate:** Also known as vitamin B9, folate is abundant in leafy greens such as spinach, kale, and Brussels sprouts.

- **Choline:** This water-soluble nutrient supports brain and nervous system function, influencing memory, mood, and muscle control. Foods like liver, eggs, soy, and broccoli are excellent sources of choline and provide antioxidant benefits.

- **Nitric Oxide:** Essential for biological processes, nitric oxide helps dilate blood vessels, improving blood flow, and reducing blood pressure and inflammation. Foods like pomegranate, beetroot, and spinach are rich in nitric oxide.

- **Probiotics and Prebiotics:** Probiotics support gut health and are found in fermented foods like yogurt and kimchi. Prebiotics, found in foods like garlic, onion, asparagus, bananas, and barley, nourish beneficial gut bacteria.

Rich Food Sources

- **Prebiotics:** Garlic, onion, asparagus, bananas, and barley.

- **Probiotics:** Yogurt, kimchi, miso, pickles (fermented), and buttermilk.

Balancing these macro and micronutrients in your diet supports daily health needs. Remember, maintaining overall health extends beyond diet—regular exercise and physical activity are equally important. The next chapter will explore incorporating these activities into your routine for optimal results.

Chapter 7:

Exercise and Physical Activity

Physical activity and exercise are foundational pillars for enhancing overall health and well-being. Whether it is taking a brisk walk in the park, tackling a challenging workout session at the gym, or indulging in a favorite sport, engaging in regular physical activity yields a multitude of benefits for both the mind and body.

This chapter will delve deeply into the profound importance of physical activity in achieving optimal health and vitality. You will explore comprehensive insights into how consistent physical activity positively impacts various aspects of your well-being, from cardiovascular health and muscular strength to mental clarity and emotional balance.

Throughout this chapter, you will uncover practical strategies and actionable tips to seamlessly integrate more movement into your daily routine. These strategies are designed to be adaptable to different lifestyles and schedules, ensuring that you can cultivate sustainable habits that promote improved health outcomes over the long term.

By embracing the significance of physical activity and incorporating it into your daily life, you will empower yourself to enhance your overall quality of life, boost energy levels, manage stress effectively, and foster a sense of well-being that extends beyond physical fitness alone.

Benefits of Regular Physical Activity

Regular physical activity has numerous benefits for both the body and the mind. Below are some of the benefits:

- **Helps Maintain a Healthy Weight:** Regular physical activity, such as exercise and physical tasks, helps balance energy consumption and expenditure, aiding in weight management. This is crucial for preventing obesity and maintaining a healthy body composition throughout life.

- **Improves Cardiovascular Health:** Physical activity strengthens the heart muscle, improves blood circulation, and reduces the risk of cardiovascular diseases such as heart disease, high blood pressure, and stroke. It also helps lower LDL (bad) cholesterol levels and raises HDL (good) cholesterol levels.

- **Boosts Mood and Mental Well-Being:** Exercise stimulates the production of endorphins, neurotransmitters that promote feelings of happiness and reduce feelings of anxiety, stress, and depression. Regular physical activity enhances overall psychological well-being and can serve as a natural mood lifter.

- **Strengthens Muscles and Bones:** Weight-bearing exercises such as resistance training and weightlifting increase muscle mass and bone density, reducing the risk of osteoporosis and improving muscular endurance and strength.

- **Enhances Flexibility and Balance:** Activities like yoga, Pilates, and stretching exercises improve flexibility, range of motion, and joint health. Balance exercises, including tai chi and specific stability drills, help reduce the risk of falls and improve overall stability, particularly important as we age.

- **Reduces the Risk of Chronic Diseases:** Regular physical activity lowers the risk of developing type 2 diabetes, certain cancers (such as breast and colon cancers), metabolic disorders, and other chronic health conditions by improving insulin sensitivity, reducing inflammation, and promoting healthy metabolic function.

- **Promotes Better Sleep Quality:** Physical activity regulates the sleep-wake cycle and promotes deeper, more restorative sleep. Regular exercise can alleviate insomnia symptoms and improve overall sleep quality, leading to better daytime alertness and cognitive function.

- **Improves Cognitive Function and Brain Health:** Exercise enhances cognitive abilities such as memory, attention, and problem-solving skills. It stimulates the release of growth factors that promote the growth of new brain cells and connections, protecting against age-related cognitive decline and reducing the risk of neurodegenerative diseases like Alzheimer's.

- **Boosts the Immune System:** Physical activity enhances immune function by promoting the circulation of immune cells throughout the body, aiding in the detection and elimination of pathogens. Regular exercise reduces the risk of infections and illnesses, contributing to overall health and well-being.

- **Increases Vitamin D Levels:** Outdoor activities, such as walking, jogging, and sports, increase exposure to sunlight and boost vitamin D levels in the body. Adequate vitamin D is essential for bone health, teeth health, muscle function, and immune system support.

- **Enhances Social Life and Relationships:** Participating in group sports, fitness classes, or community exercise programs fosters social interaction and camaraderie. Building relationships through physical activity reduces feelings of loneliness, and promotes teamwork, communication, and interpersonal skills.

- **Ensures Well-Rounded Fitness:** Incorporating a variety of exercises into your routine ensures well-rounded physical fitness, including cardiovascular exercises (e.g., running, cycling), strength training (e.g., weightlifting, bodyweight exercises), flexibility workouts (e.g., yoga, stretching), and relaxation techniques (e.g., meditation, deep breathing). This approach supports overall health, balance, coordination, and agility, preventing fitness plateaus and promoting lifelong physical well-being.

These benefits highlight the holistic advantages of integrating physical activity into daily life for improved health outcomes.

Types of Exercises for Different Age Groups

Regular physical activity is essential for people of all ages to maintain their overall health and well-being. Tailoring exercise routines to specific age groups helps ensure that the exercises are safe, effective, and enjoyable. Different age groups have different needs and capabilities, so targeted exercises can promote optimal health and fitness levels accordingly. Understanding the appropriate types of exercises for various age groups is crucial in helping individuals enhance their quality of life through regular physical activity.

Here are the types of exercises suitable for different age groups:

Children and Adolescents

- **Active Play:** Encourages running, jumping, and playing sports to enhance physical fitness, coordination, and social skills. It is vital for developing motor skills and learning teamwork.

- **Swimming:** Provides a full-body workout that improves cardiovascular fitness, endurance, and muscle strength. It is particularly beneficial as it is low-impact, making it suitable for children with joint issues.

- **Gymnastics:** Develops flexibility, strength, coordination, and body awareness through activities like tumbling, balancing, and vaulting. It enhances agility and motor control.

- **Outdoor Exploration:** Engages children in nature, fostering curiosity about ecosystems and wildlife. It promotes physical activity while teaching environmental appreciation and stewardship.

- **Dance Classes:** Combines fun with physical activity, boosting creativity, rhythm, and cardiovascular fitness. Dance classes improve coordination, flexibility, and self-expression.

- **Yoga:** Teaches mindfulness, balance, and relaxation techniques through poses and breathing exercises. It enhances flexibility, body awareness, and mental well-being from a young age.

- **Sports Teams:** Fosters teamwork, discipline, and sportsmanship in a competitive setting. Participation in sports like soccer, basketball, or baseball promotes physical fitness, strategic thinking, and social skills development.

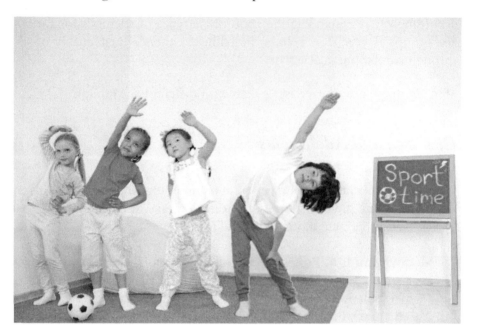

Adults

- **Cardiovascular Exercises:** Running, cycling, and aerobics improve heart health, stamina, and calorie burning. These activities boost cardiovascular fitness, enhance endurance, and contribute to weight management.

- **Strength Training:** Involves weightlifting or bodyweight exercises to build muscle mass, maintain bone density, and increase metabolism. It enhances strength, improves posture, and supports joint health.

- **Yoga:** Enhances flexibility, balance, stress management, and overall well-being through various poses and relaxation techniques. Yoga promotes mindfulness, reduces stress levels, and improves mental focus.

- **Swimming:** Offers a full-body workout that enhances cardiovascular health, muscle tone, and endurance. It is gentle on joints and suitable for all fitness levels, making it ideal for both leisure and fitness purposes.

- **Pilates:** Focuses on core strength, stability, flexibility, posture, and muscle control through controlled movements and breathing techniques. It improves muscle tone, enhances flexibility, and supports spinal health.

- **HIIT (High-Intensity Interval Training):** Provides quick, efficient workouts alternating between intense bursts of activity and short recovery periods. HIIT improves cardiovascular fitness, boosts metabolism, and burns calories effectively.

- **Piloxing:** Combines Pilates and boxing for a dynamic workout that enhances strength, agility, coordination, and cardiovascular health. It provides a full-body workout while incorporating elements of dance and martial arts.

- **CrossFit:** Incorporates diverse functional movements like lifting, pushing, and pulling to improve strength, cardiovascular fitness, and overall physical performance. It promotes agility, power, and endurance through high-intensity workouts.

- **Dance Fitness:** Uses dance movements and aerobic exercises to improve coordination, cardiovascular health, and mood. It is a fun way to exercise while enhancing rhythm, flexibility, and overall fitness.

- **Hiking:** Offers outdoor enjoyment while providing cardiovascular benefits, muscle toning, and stress relief. Hiking improves endurance, strengthens lower body muscles, and promotes mental relaxation through nature exploration.

- **Kickboxing:** Combines martial arts techniques with cardio exercises to tone muscles, improve cardiovascular health, and release stress. It enhances agility, coordination, and core strength while providing a high-energy workout.

- **TRX Suspension Training:** Uses suspension straps and bodyweight exercises to strengthen muscles, improve stability, and enhance core strength. It is adaptable for all fitness levels and focuses on functional strength and flexibility.

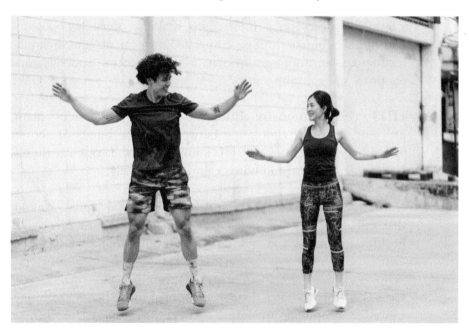

Older Adults

- **Walking:** Improves cardiovascular health, muscle strength, and joint flexibility with minimal impact on joints. Walking is accessible, promotes bone density, and enhances overall mobility and endurance.

- **Tai Chi:** Promotes balance, coordination, and relaxation, and reduces fall risk through slow, deliberate movements and deep breathing exercises. It enhances flexibility, mental clarity, and overall well-being.

- **Water Aerobics:** Gentle on joints, water aerobics maintains muscle mass, improves flexibility, and supports cardiovascular health through water resistance exercises. It is beneficial for arthritis management and overall fitness.

- **Yoga:** Enhances balance, flexibility, and mental well-being through gentle poses and breathing exercises tailored for older adults. Yoga improves posture, reduces stress levels, and promotes relaxation and mindfulness.

- **Dancing:** Provides enjoyment while improving balance, cognitive function, and overall fitness. Dancing enhances coordination, promotes social interaction, and boosts mood and self-esteem among older adults.

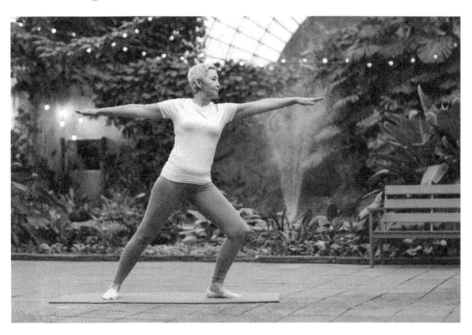

These exercises are tailored to each age group's specific physical abilities and needs, promoting overall health, fitness, and well-being throughout life.

Tips for Incorporating Exercise Into Daily Routine

Incorporating exercise into your daily routine is crucial for maintaining overall health and well-being. By prioritizing physical activity daily, you can improve your fitness levels, boost your mood, and enhance your quality of life. Here are seven tips to help you seamlessly integrate exercise into your daily schedule:

Setting Realistic Goals:	Define specific and achievable fitness objectives that match your fitness level and lifestyle. Gradually increase workout intensity and duration to challenge yourself while staying motivated. Celebrate small achievements to track progress and maintain inspiration.
Scheduling Workouts:	Treat exercise as a priority by scheduling it into your daily calendar. Block out dedicated time slots for workouts, choosing your most convenient and least busy times to ensure commitment without distractions. Prioritizing exercise in your schedule underscores its importance for your health and well-being.
Mixing It Up:	Prevent boredom and target different muscle groups by engaging in various exercises. Include cardiovascular activities, strength training, flexibility exercises, and enjoyable physical activities like dancing or recreational sports. Experiment with new workout classes or outdoor activities to keep your routine stimulating and challenging.
Finding Enjoyable Activities:	Select exercises you genuinely enjoy to sustain long-term commitment. Whether it is dancing, swimming, hiking, or playing a sport you love, incorporating enjoyable activities makes exercise feel rewarding rather than a chore. Explore different forms of physical activity to find what fits best into your lifestyle.

Creating Accountability:	Work out with a friend, join a fitness class, or hire a personal trainer for accountability and support. Sharing workouts with others makes exercise more enjoyable and motivating. A trainer can provide guidance and motivation to help you surpass limits and achieve fitness goals, ensuring consistency and dedication.
Incorporating Short Workouts:	Boost overall activity levels by integrating short bursts of physical activity throughout your day. Opt for the stairs instead of the elevator, do quick exercises during TV commercials, or take brisk walks during breaks. These mini-sessions add to daily physical activity, enhance energy levels, improve mood, and break sedentary habits.
Prioritizing Recovery:	Rest and recovery are essential for a balanced fitness routine. Schedule rest days to allow your body time to repair muscles, prevent overtraining, and reduce injury risk. Ensure adequate sleep, proper nutrition, and hydration to support muscle recovery and overall well-being. Prioritizing recovery ensures sustainable enjoyment of your exercise routine.

Exercise and physical activity offer numerous benefits, including weight management, improved cardiovascular health, mood enhancement, and reduced chronic disease risk. Tailoring exercises to different age groups promotes optimal health and fitness levels. Understanding the importance of staying active and incorporating diverse exercises contributes to a balanced lifestyle.

In the next chapter, we will explore the impact of social connections and emotional well-being on health, along with ways to nurture them for a fulfilling life.

Chapter 8:

Social Connections and Emotional

Well-Being

In this chapter, we will explore the significance of social relationships for your health and well-being. You will discover why fostering meaningful connections and nurturing your emotional well-being are crucial components of a fulfilling life.

Social relationships play a vital role in our lives, impacting our physical health, mental well-being, and overall quality of life. Research consistently shows that strong social ties can contribute to longevity, reduced risk of chronic diseases, and faster recovery from illness. Beyond the physical benefits, meaningful connections provide emotional support, reduce feelings of loneliness and isolation, and enhance our sense of belonging and purpose.

Throughout this chapter, we will examine various strategies and insights to help you cultivate and maintain positive social connections. You will learn practical tips on how to strengthen existing relationships and build new ones, regardless of your age or circumstances. From effective communication skills to nurturing empathy and understanding, these strategies will empower you to create deeper, more meaningful bonds with others.

Additionally, we will discuss the importance of nurturing your emotional health. Emotional well-being is essential for managing stress, coping with challenges, and maintaining a positive outlook on life. You will discover actionable techniques to enhance your emotional resilience, such as mindfulness practices, self-care routines, and seeking support when needed.

By understanding the impact of social relationships and emotional well-being on your overall strength and resilience, you will be equipped to cultivate a supportive network and lead a more fulfilling life. Together, let us explore how staying connected with others and prioritizing your emotional health can enrich your journey toward holistic well-being.

Impact of Social Interactions on Health

Social interactions profoundly influence an individual's physical, mental, and emotional well-being, playing a pivotal role in promoting overall wellness across several key areas:

- **Mental Health:** Strong social connections are essential for maintaining good mental health. Engaging in meaningful conversations and receiving support from others can alleviate feelings of loneliness, stress, and anxiety. This support network helps reduce the risk of developing depression and mood disorders by providing emotional stability and a sense of belonging.

- **Emotional Well-Being:** Positive social interactions contribute to feelings of happiness, contentment, and fulfillment. Sharing experiences and emotions, and receiving support from friends and family members enhance emotional resilience. During challenging times, these interactions bolster coping skills, providing a source of strength and comfort.

- **Physical Health:** Surprisingly, social ties significantly impact physical health outcomes. Individuals with robust relationships tend to experience lower rates of chronic diseases, faster recovery from illnesses, and increased longevity. Engaging in social activities has been linked to lower blood pressure, improved immune function, and overall better physical well-being.

- **Stress Reduction:** Social interactions act as a buffer against stress by providing emotional support and promoting relaxation. Spending time with supportive individuals or participating in group activities helps manage stress levels effectively. This support network enhances resilience, enabling individuals to navigate stressful situations with greater ease.

- **Cognitive Function:** Social engagement stimulates cognitive function and promotes brain health. Active discussions, social interactions, and participating in group activities stimulate the brain, improving memory, cognitive skills, and overall mental agility. These activities may potentially lower the risk of cognitive decline associated with aging.

- **Behavioral Patterns:** Social connections influence behavior and lifestyle choices. Being part of a supportive community encourages healthy habits such as regular exercise, balanced nutrition, and positive coping strategies. By fostering these behaviors, social networks contribute to long-term physical and mental well-being.

- **Sense of Purpose:** Meaningful social interactions provide a sense of purpose and belonging. Being connected to others and actively involved in a community fosters a sense of identity and fulfillment. This sense of purpose contributes to overall life satisfaction, promoting a positive outlook and enhancing mental resilience.

Recognizing the profound impact of social interactions, individuals can prioritize building and nurturing meaningful relationships in their lives. By actively engaging in social activities, maintaining close connections, and seeking out support networks, people can enhance their holistic well-being and resilience. Investing in these relationships fosters a happier, healthier life, characterized by emotional strength, physical vitality, and a sense of fulfillment.

Building and Maintaining Social Connections

Building and maintaining social connections is vital for fostering meaningful relationships, promoting emotional well-being, and enhancing overall quality of life. Cultivating strong social ties requires effort, effective communication, and a genuine interest in connecting with others. Here are key strategies to help you build and maintain social connections:

- **Open Communication:** Establish trust and understanding by being open, honest, and transparent in your interactions. Actively listen to others, share your thoughts and feelings, and empathize with their perspectives. Effective communication strengthens interpersonal bonds and fosters deeper connections.

- **Initiate Interactions:** Take proactive steps to reach out and engage with others. Invite friends for coffee or meals, attend social gatherings, join clubs, or participate in community events where you can meet new people. Stepping out of your comfort zone and initiating interactions is essential for expanding your social circle and building new connections.

- **Maintain Consistency:** Nurture relationships over time by staying in touch regularly. Simple gestures like phone calls, texts, or social media interactions help maintain connections and demonstrate your care and interest in others' lives. Consistency in communication reinforces the strength of your relationships.

- **Quality Over Quantity:** Focus on nurturing close friendships and meaningful connections with individuals who share similar values, interests, and goals. Quality relationships provide emotional support, mutual trust, and a sense of belonging, enhancing overall well-being and satisfaction.

- **Be Authentic:** Build genuine connections by being true to yourself in your interactions. Share your thoughts, feelings, and experiences honestly, and show vulnerability when appropriate. Authenticity fosters deeper connections based on mutual respect and understanding, laying the foundation for meaningful relationships.

- **Be Supportive:** Strengthen bonds by offering encouragement, comfort, and celebration during both challenging times and moments of success. Being a supportive presence in others' lives builds trust and reciprocity, deepening your connections and fostering a supportive social network.

- **Shared Activities:** Bond with others through shared hobbies, sports activities, group outings, or volunteer opportunities. Engaging in shared experiences creates opportunities for meaningful interactions, builds camaraderie, and strengthens relationships through shared memories and interests.

- **Respect Boundaries:** Honor the preferences, personal space, and time of others in your social interactions. Communicate openly about expectations in the relationship, and respect their boundaries and privacy. Mutual respect fosters healthier and more sustainable connections over time.

- **Celebrate Diversity:** Embrace and appreciate the unique qualities, backgrounds, and perspectives of individuals from diverse cultures and experiences. Building connections across different backgrounds enriches social interactions, promotes mutual learning, and enhances empathy and understanding.

By integrating these strategies into your daily interactions and relationships, you can cultivate strong social connections that enrich your life, provide support during difficult times, and contribute to your overall well-being and happiness. Investing in meaningful relationships fosters a sense of community, belonging, and emotional fulfillment, enhancing both your personal and social spheres of life.

Strategies for Enhancing Emotional Well-Being

Enhancing emotional well-being is crucial for maintaining good mental health, resilience, and overall quality of life. By incorporating effective strategies into daily routines, individuals can cultivate emotional strength, self-awareness, and coping mechanisms to navigate challenges and promote well-being. Here are key strategies for enhancing emotional well-being:

- **Mindfulness and Meditation:** Practicing mindfulness involves being fully present in the moment, observing thoughts and emotions without judgment, and cultivating self-awareness. Meditation techniques such as deep breathing, body scans, and guided meditation sessions help reduce stress, promote relaxation, and improve emotional balance by calming the mind and increasing awareness of inner experiences.

- **Emotional Expression:** Healthy emotional expression is essential for processing and managing feelings effectively. Find outlets such as journaling, talking openly to a trusted friend or therapist, engaging in creative activities like art or music, or participating in mindfulness-based therapies like cognitive-behavioral therapy (CBT). These practices allow for the acknowledgment and exploration of emotions, facilitating healing, and personal growth.

- **Physical Activity:** Regular exercise is a powerful tool for enhancing emotional well-being. Physical activity releases endorphins, serotonin, and dopamine—natural chemicals that elevate mood, reduce stress levels, and promote a sense of well-being. Activities such as walking, running, yoga, or dancing not only improve physical health but also boost emotional resilience and overall mental health.

- **Healthy Lifestyle Choices:** Adopting healthy habits such as maintaining balanced nutrition, getting adequate sleep, and avoiding excessive substances like alcohol and drugs is crucial for emotional stability and resilience. A healthy body supports a healthy mind, enhancing the ability to cope with stress and maintain emotional balance.

- **Self-Care Practices:** Prioritizing self-care activities that bring joy, relaxation, and fulfillment is vital for emotional well-being. Engage in activities such as reading, taking soothing baths, spending time outdoors in nature, or practicing relaxation techniques like deep breathing or progressive muscle relaxation. Setting boundaries, practicing self-compassion, and nurturing oneself physically, emotionally, and mentally are essential components of effective self-care.

- **Social Support:** Building and maintaining strong social connections provide vital emotional support during challenging times and foster a sense of belonging and community. Seek support from friends and family members, or participate in support groups where you can share experiences, receive encouragement, and reduce feelings of loneliness and isolation.

- **Stress Management:** Developing effective stress management techniques is crucial for maintaining emotional balance. Practice relaxation methods such as deep breathing exercises, mindfulness meditation, or progressive muscle relaxation (PMR) to reduce physiological arousal and manage stress levels effectively. Time management strategies and setting priorities can also help alleviate stress and promote emotional well-being.

- **Gratitude Practices:** Cultivating a practice of gratitude can significantly enhance emotional well-being by shifting focus toward positive aspects of life. Consider keeping a gratitude journal where you regularly write down things you are thankful for or express appreciation to others. Gratitude promotes a positive mindset, enhances resilience, and fosters emotional well-being.

- **Mind-Body Connection:** Acknowledging and nurturing the connection between the mind and body is essential for holistic emotional health. Engage in practices like yoga, tai chi, or aromatherapy that promote relaxation, reduce stress, and restore balance to both mental and physical well-being.

- **Professional Support:** Seek help from mental health professionals such as therapists, counselors, or psychologists when needed. Professional support provides valuable insights, coping strategies, and interventions for managing emotional challenges and promoting overall well-being.

Incorporating these strategies into daily routines enhances emotional well-being, builds resilience, and fosters a positive outlook on life. By nurturing emotional health through mindfulness, healthy habits, social connections, and self-care practices, individuals can effectively manage stress, navigate life's challenges, and cultivate a sense of fulfillment and happiness.

The next chapter will delve into the profound significance of quality sleep in the context of healthy aging. It will explore how prioritizing good sleep hygiene and effectively managing sleep disorders can significantly enhance overall well-being as we age. It will also share practical tips and strategies to improve sleep hygiene.

Chapter 9:

Sleep and Rest

Adequate and quality sleep is fundamental to maintaining overall health, vitality, and cognitive function, especially as we age. On the path to healthy aging, the importance of restorative sleep cannot be overstated. It plays a critical role in physical recovery, mental clarity, emotional stability, and immune function. As we grow older, changes in sleep patterns and the prevalence of sleep disorders can significantly impact our quality of life. Therefore, prioritizing sleep and implementing effective strategies to improve sleep hygiene is essential.

This chapter delves into the crucial role of quality sleep in promoting healthy aging, exploring tips to enhance sleep hygiene and strategies to manage common sleep disorders effectively. By understanding the importance of proper sleep habits and addressing sleep-related challenges, individuals can optimize their rest patterns and support their well-being for a fulfilling and vibrant life ahead. Let us uncover the key aspects of sleep and rest contributing to healthy aging and well-being.

Importance of Quality Sleep for Healthy Aging

To age gracefully and maintain overall well-being, quality sleep plays a crucial role. The influence of sleep on diverse aspects of health—ranging from cognitive function and emotional stability to physical well-being—is profound. Adequate and restful sleep supports the body's natural repair processes, enhances memory consolidation, and regulates emotions. As individuals navigate the journey of aging, prioritizing quality sleep becomes a cornerstone in fostering vitality, resilience, and a thriving quality of life. Below are some key points on the importance of quality sleep for healthy aging:

- **Cognitive Function:** Quality sleep enhances brain function, making it easier to learn new information, retain knowledge, and think clearly. When well-rested, the brain operates optimally, enabling individuals to tackle tasks requiring significant cognitive effort without feeling mentally fatigued.

- **Emotional Well-Being:** Restful sleep is vital for emotional regulation. Adequate sleep helps in managing emotions, reducing stress levels, and maintaining a balanced mood. By ensuring sufficient rest, individuals can experience greater emotional stability, which is crucial for overall mental health and well-being.

- **Physical Health:** Quality sleep supports physical health in several ways. It facilitates cellular repair processes, strengthens the immune system, and ensures optimal functioning of bodily systems. This contributes to overall physical health and vitality, providing the energy necessary for engaging in daily activities and pursuing hobbies.

- **Metabolic Health:** Good quality sleep plays a significant role in metabolic health. It helps regulate appetite hormones, such as leptin and ghrelin, which control hunger and satiety. Consistent sleep patterns support efficient energy utilization and metabolism, reducing the risk of metabolic disorders such as diabetes and obesity.

- **Longevity:** Regular, quality sleep is essential for long-term health and longevity. It boosts the immune system, lowers inflammation levels, and decreases the likelihood of developing chronic illnesses. By promoting overall health and resilience, quality sleep contributes to a longer and healthier life span.

Incorporating practices that prioritize sleep hygiene, such as maintaining a consistent sleep schedule, creating a relaxing bedtime routine, and ensuring a conducive sleep environment, can significantly enhance these benefits. Prioritizing quality sleep is not just about feeling refreshed—it is a cornerstone of maintaining optimal health across the lifespan.

Tips for Improving Sleep Hygiene

Improving sleep hygiene is essential for enhancing the quality of your sleep and overall well-being. By incorporating simple yet effective practices into your daily routine, you can create a conducive environment for restful and rejuvenating sleep. These tips focus on establishing healthy habits that promote relaxation, comfort, and consistency to optimize your sleep hygiene.

- **Establish a Consistent Sleep Schedule:** This is crucial for training your body's internal clock and improving overall sleep quality. By setting a regular bedtime and wake-up time, you synchronize your sleep-wake cycle, helping your body know when it is time to rest and when to wake up naturally. Consistency in your sleep schedule enhances sleep efficiency and promotes deeper, more restorative sleep each night.

- **Create a Relaxing Bedtime Routine:** This enhances your ability to unwind and prepare for sleep effectively. Engaging in calming activities before bed signals to your body that it is time to wind down. Activities such as reading a book, taking a warm bath, or practicing relaxation techniques like deep breathing can help reduce stress and ease your mind from the day's demands. Establishing a bedtime routine trains your body to recognize sleep cues and transition into a state of relaxation conducive to falling asleep easily.

- **Ensure Your Bedroom Is Sleep-Conducive:** This involves optimizing your sleep environment to promote uninterrupted rest. Your bedroom should be quiet, dark, and cool to create an ideal setting for sleep. Consider using earplugs or a white noise machine to block out disruptive sounds, and blackout curtains to eliminate light disturbances that can interfere with your sleep cycle. Creating a peaceful sleep environment enhances your ability to achieve deep, restful sleep throughout the night.

- **Limit Screen Time Before Bed:** Doing that is essential for minimizing the impact of blue light exposure on your sleep quality. The blue light emitted from screens can suppress melatonin production, making it harder to fall asleep. To promote better sleep hygiene, limit screen use at least an hour before bedtime. If you must use screens close to bedtime, consider using blue light filters or apps that reduce blue light emission to mitigate its effects on your sleep-wake cycle.

- **Manage Stress Throughout the Day:** This is crucial for promoting relaxation and reducing sleep disturbances. Engaging in stress-relieving activities such as exercise, meditation, or spending time outdoors can help alleviate tension and prepare your mind and body for sleep. By addressing stressors earlier in the day, you can promote a sense of calm and relaxation at bedtime, enhancing your ability to fall asleep and stay asleep throughout the night.

- **Watch Your Diet and Hydration:** That plays a significant role in promoting healthy sleep patterns. Avoid consuming heavy meals and caffeine close to bedtime, as these can disrupt your sleep and cause nighttime awakenings. Opt for light, nutritious snacks if you are hungry before bed, and stay hydrated throughout the day to prevent sleep disturbances caused by thirst. Maintaining a balanced diet and adequate hydration supports overall health and contributes to better sleep quality.

- **Get Regular Exercise:** Doing this is beneficial for improving sleep quality and promoting restorative sleep. Engaging in at least 30 minutes of moderate physical activity most days of the week can help regulate your sleep-wake cycle and enhance your ability to fall asleep quickly and stay asleep longer. However, avoid vigorous exercise close to bedtime, as it may energize your body and make it more difficult to wind down for sleep.

- **Optimize Your Sleep Environment:** This involves creating a comfortable and supportive setting that promotes restful sleep. Investing in a high-quality mattress and pillows that provide adequate support can enhance your sleep comfort and reduce discomfort that may disrupt sleep. Ensure your sleep space is free of allergens and other irritants that could affect your breathing and sleep quality. A well-designed sleep environment contributes to a restorative sleep experience and improves overall sleep satisfaction.

- **Wind Down Before Bedtime:** This is essential for preparing your mind and body for sleep. Establishing a calming bedtime routine that includes relaxing activities helps signal to your body that it is time to wind down and prepare for rest. Avoid stimulating activities and screens during this time, opting instead for activities that promote relaxation and tranquility. By cultivating a consistent bedtime routine, you can optimize your sleep quality and promote a seamless transition into restful sleep each night.

- **Seek Professional Help if Needed:** This is important if you continue to experience sleep problems despite implementing these strategies. Consulting a healthcare provider or sleep specialist can provide personalized evaluation and recommendations tailored to address underlying sleep issues. They can conduct a thorough assessment to identify any medical conditions contributing to sleep disturbances and recommend appropriate treatments, such as medications or cognitive-behavioral therapy for insomnia, to help you achieve better sleep quality and overall well-being.

Strategies for Managing Sleep Disorders

Sleep disorders can arise from various factors, with stress and anxiety being common contributors. When individuals are anxious or worried, their minds can become restless, making it challenging to fall or stay asleep. Poor sleep habits, such as irregular sleep schedules or excessive screen time before bed, disrupt the body's natural sleep-wake cycle and contribute to sleep disorders. Additionally, medical conditions like sleep apnea, insomnia, or restless leg syndrome can significantly impact sleep quality.

- **Coping Mechanisms for Stress and Anxiety:** Managing sleep disorders caused by stress and anxiety involves adopting coping mechanisms that promote relaxation. Techniques such as deep breathing exercises, mindfulness meditation, or progressive muscle relaxation (PMR) can calm the mind and body before bedtime. Establishing a soothing bedtime routine, like reading a book or taking a warm bath, signals to the body that it is time to transition into sleep mode.

- **Improving Sleep Hygiene:** Developing good sleep hygiene practices is crucial for those struggling with sleep disorders. Consistently following a sleep schedule where bedtime and wake-up times are consistent helps regulate the body's internal clock and enhances sleep quality. Avoiding stimulants such as caffeine and nicotine close to bedtime and creating a sleep-friendly environment—dark, quiet, and comfortably cool—promotes better sleep.

- **The Role of Diet and Exercise:** Maintaining a healthy diet and regular exercise routine positively influences sleep patterns. Consuming heavy or spicy meals late in the day can cause discomfort and disrupt sleep while opting for light, nutritious snacks can aid digestion and promote better rest. Engaging in physical activity earlier in the day reduces stress and promotes relaxation, contributing to improved sleep quality.

- **Seeking Professional Help:** Persistent sleep disorders may necessitate seeking help from a healthcare professional. A doctor can conduct a comprehensive evaluation to identify underlying medical conditions contributing to sleep disturbances. They may recommend treatments such as medication and cognitive-behavioral therapy for insomnia, or refer individuals to a sleep specialist for further assessment.

- **Support From Sleep Specialists:** Sleep specialists possess expertise in diagnosing and treating various sleep disorders. Consulting a sleep specialist allows individuals to receive personalized treatment plans tailored to their specific needs. These specialists may recommend specific behavioral adjustments, prescribe medications if necessary, or suggest alternative therapies to enhance sleep quality and overall well-being.In this chapter, we have thoroughly examined the role of sleep and rest in maintaining overall health. The next chapter will discuss methods for managing chronic conditions.

Chapter 10:

Managing Chronic Conditions

As individuals age, they commonly experience persistent health issues. Research indicates that nearly every adult over 60 years old deals with at least one chronic condition, with a majority managing two or more (Silberman, 2022). Obesity emerges as a significant contributor, substantially raising the risk of conditions such as diabetes, heart disease, and cancer, affecting approximately 42% of adults aged 60 and above (Bryan et al., 2021).

Among Medicare beneficiaries aged 65 and older, the most prevalent conditions treated include high blood pressure, high cholesterol, obesity, arthritis, heart disease, kidney problems, heart failure, depression, Alzheimer's disease, and dementia (Silberman, 2022). Each of these conditions poses distinct challenges and necessitates tailored approaches to management and prevention.

This chapter aims to delve into effective strategies for addressing chronic conditions in older adults. By exploring comprehensive management techniques and preventive measures, it seeks to empower individuals and healthcare providers alike in optimizing health outcomes and enhancing quality of life in aging populations.

Hypertension

Hypertension, or high blood pressure, is a prevalent medical condition characterized by elevated blood pressure levels, where the force of blood against the artery walls is abnormally high. This persistent condition can gradually damage blood vessels and vital organs such as the heart, brain, kidneys, and eyes, increasing the risk of serious health complications like heart disease, stroke, and kidney failure over time. Despite its potential severity, hypertension is often asymptomatic, earning it the nickname "silent killer" because individuals may not be aware of the condition until significant damage has occurred.

In adults, blood pressure is typically measured using two numbers:

- Systolic pressure, the higher number, represents the pressure in the arteries when the heart beats and pumps blood.

- Diastolic pressure, the lower number, indicates the pressure in the arteries when the heart rests between beats.

Normal blood pressure for adults is generally defined as a systolic pressure of 120 or less and a diastolic pressure of 80 or less. When blood pressure readings consistently fall between 120-129 systolic and less than 80 diastolic, individuals are classified as having elevated blood pressure. Hypertension is diagnosed when systolic blood pressure reaches 130 or higher and/or diastolic blood pressure is 80 or higher.

Risk Factors for Hypertension

Risk factors for developing hypertension encompass a variety of influences:

- **Age:** The risk of hypertension increases with age.

- **Family History:** Hypertension often runs in families, suggesting a genetic predisposition.

- **Weight:** Being overweight or obese significantly elevates the risk of developing high blood pressure.

- **Physical Inactivity:** Lack of regular physical activity is associated with higher blood pressure levels.

- **Diet:** Consuming a diet high in sodium, low in potassium, and excessive in alcohol can contribute to the development of hypertension.

- **Tobacco Use:** Smoking or using tobacco products raises blood pressure temporarily and can damage artery walls over time.

- **Stress:** Chronic stress can lead to temporary spikes in blood pressure.

- **Chronic Conditions:** Conditions like diabetes and kidney disease increase the likelihood of hypertension.

Understanding these risk factors can help individuals make informed lifestyle choices and seek early intervention to prevent or manage hypertension effectively.

Tips to Manage and Prevent Hypertension

Managing and preventing high blood pressure involves adopting several beneficial lifestyle changes and habits that can easily fit into your daily routine:

- **Adopt a Balanced Diet:** Start by monitoring your salt intake, aiming for less than 2,300 milligrams per day (about one teaspoon). Ideally, reducing it further is even better. Increase consumption of potassium-rich foods like bananas, oranges, and spinach, as potassium helps counteract the effects of sodium. Emphasize a diet rich in fruits, vegetables, whole grains, and lean proteins to support overall health.

- **Exercise Regularly:** Maintaining an active lifestyle is crucial. Aim for at least moderate-intensity exercise most days of the week, such as brisk walking, swimming, or dancing. Incorporate strength training activities like weight lifting or resistance exercises to add variety and effectiveness to your workout routine.

- **Manage Weight:** If you are carrying extra weight, even modest weight loss can have a significant impact on lowering blood pressure. Focus on making sustainable changes to your diet and exercise habits rather than drastic measures.

- **Monitor Blood Pressure:** Regularly checking your blood pressure with your healthcare provider is essential for managing hypertension. Consider using a home blood pressure monitor to track your levels between medical appointments and to stay informed about your health status.

- **Reduce Stress:** Effective stress management techniques can help lower blood pressure. Practice relaxation methods such as deep breathing, meditation, or yoga. Engage in hobbies and activities you enjoy, and prioritize spending time with loved ones to promote emotional well-being.

- **Quit Smoking and Moderate Alcohol:** If you smoke, quitting is one of the most impactful steps you can take for your overall health, including lowering blood pressure. Seek support and resources to help you quit successfully. Limit alcohol intake to moderate levels—up to one drink per day for women and up to two for men—since excessive alcohol consumption can raise blood pressure levels.

By incorporating these lifestyle changes and habits into your daily life, you can effectively manage high blood pressure and improve your overall health and well-being.

Type 2 Diabetes

Type 2 diabetes is a chronic condition that affects how the body processes blood sugar (glucose). Unlike type 1 diabetes, which involves the body's inability to produce insulin, type 2 diabetes is primarily characterized by insulin resistance. In this condition, the body's cells do not respond effectively to insulin, leading to elevated levels of blood sugar. If left unmanaged, these high blood sugar levels can result in various health complications.

Risk Factors for Type 2 Diabetes

Several factors can increase the risk of developing type 2 diabetes, including:

- **Age:** The risk tends to increase with age, particularly after 45 years old.

- **Family History:** Having a parent or sibling with type 2 diabetes increases your risk.

- **Weight:** Being overweight or obese, especially if you carry excess fat around your abdomen.

- **Physical Inactivity:** Not engaging in regular physical activities raises the risk.

- **Diet:** Consuming a diet high in processed foods, sugary beverages, and unhealthy fats can increase the risk.

- **Ethnicity:** Certain ethnic groups, including African Americans, Hispanics, Native Americans, and Asian Americans, have a higher risk.

- **High Blood Pressure:** Hypertension (high blood pressure) is associated with an increased risk of developing type 2 diabetes.

Tips to Slow or Prevent the Onset of Type 2 Diabetes

To slow or prevent the onset of type 2 diabetes, consider adopting the following strategies:

- **Eat Healthy:** Focus on consuming more whole grains, fruits, vegetables, lean proteins, and healthy fats. Reduce intake of sugary drinks, sweets, and refined grains. Pay attention to portion sizes to avoid overeating.

- **Exercise Regularly:** Aim for at least 150 minutes of moderate-intensity aerobic exercise per week, such as walking, swimming, or cycling. Incorporate strength training exercises at least twice a week to build muscle and improve insulin sensitivity.

- **Manage Your Weight:** Strive to maintain a healthy weight through a balanced diet and regular exercise. Even modest weight loss can significantly lower the risk of developing diabetes.

- **Monitor Regularly:** If you are at risk, monitor your blood sugar levels regularly. Schedule regular checkups with your doctor to assess your overall health and detect any early signs of diabetes.

- **Practice Relaxation Techniques:** Engage in activities like yoga, meditation, or deep-breathing exercises to manage stress levels, which can impact blood sugar regulation. Stress management is crucial for maintaining overall well-being and reducing diabetes risk.

High Cholesterol

High cholesterol is common among seniors, characterized by an accumulation of excess bad fats or lipids in the body. These lipids can build up in arteries, leading to blockages that increase the risk of heart disease.

Risk Factors for High Cholesterol

Several factors can contribute to elevated cholesterol levels:

- **Diet:** Consuming excessive saturated fats, commonly found in foods like butter, cheese, and fatty meats, can increase cholesterol levels.

- **Weight:** Being overweight or obese can also elevate cholesterol levels.

- **Physical Activity:** Insufficient exercise can lower HDL (good) cholesterol levels and raise LDL (bad) cholesterol levels.

- **Age and Gender:** Cholesterol levels typically increase with age, and men tend to have higher cholesterol levels before the age of 50.

- **Family History:** A family history of high cholesterol can predispose individuals to elevated cholesterol levels.

Tips to Prevent or Manage High Cholesterol

Here are effective strategies for preventing or managing high cholesterol:

- **Include Fiber-Rich Foods:** Incorporate foods high in soluble fiber, such as oats, legumes (like beans and lentils), and certain fruits (like apples and oranges). Soluble fiber helps lower LDL cholesterol levels.

- **Choose Healthy Fats:** Opt for healthier fats like mono- and polyunsaturated fats found in olive oil, avocados, nuts (such as almonds and walnuts), and fatty fish (like salmon and trout). These fats can improve your cholesterol profile by raising HDL cholesterol and lowering LDL cholesterol.

- **Prioritize Quality Sleep:** Aim for 7-9 hours of quality sleep each night. Poor sleep patterns can negatively impact cholesterol levels and overall health.

- **Stay Hydrated:** Drinking enough water supports the proper metabolism of fats and cholesterol. Aim for at least 8 glasses (about 2 liters) of water daily to maintain overall health, including cholesterol management.

Obesity

Obesity is characterized by an excessive accumulation of body fat that can significantly impact health. It extends beyond simply being overweight, representing a chronic disease associated with various health conditions. These include hypertension, type 2 diabetes, dyslipidemia, cerebral vasculopathy, sleep apnea, and numerous others (De Lorenzo et al., 2019).

Risk Factors for Obesity

Several factors contribute to the development of obesity:

- **Unhealthy Diet:** Consuming excessive calories, especially from fast food, sugary beverages, and large portions, can lead to weight gain.

- **Sedentary Lifestyle:** Lack of physical activity or prolonged periods of inactivity contribute to weight gain.

- **Genetics:** Family history and genetic predisposition can influence an individual's likelihood of developing obesity.

- **Emotional Factors:** Stress, inadequate sleep, and emotional eating behaviors can lead to overeating and weight gain.

- **Medical Conditions:** Certain medical conditions and medications may promote weight gain or hinder weight loss efforts.

Tips to Prevent or Manage Obesity

Here are effective strategies to prevent or manage obesity:

- **Adopt a Balanced Diet and Portion Control:** Emphasize whole, unprocessed foods such as fruits, vegetables, lean proteins, and whole grains. Avoid large portions, especially of high-calorie foods.

- **Increase Physical Activity:** Incorporate regular indoor and outdoor physical activities to avoid a sedentary lifestyle.

- **Seek Support:** Consider joining a weight-loss group or consulting with healthcare professionals such as registered dietitians or fitness trainers to help achieve your goals.

Arthritis

Arthritis is a condition characterized by joint pain, stiffness, and inflammation, which can significantly impact daily life and reduce overall quality of life. The two most common types of arthritis are osteoarthritis and rheumatoid arthritis.

Risk Factors for Arthritis

Several factors contribute to an increased risk of developing arthritis:

- **Age:** The likelihood of developing arthritis, particularly osteoarthritis, increases with age.

- **Gender:** Women are more susceptible to rheumatoid arthritis, whereas men are more prone to gout.

- **Family History:** Genetics play a role in predisposing individuals to various forms of arthritis.

- **Occupational Hazards:** Jobs involving repetitive movements or heavy lifting can heighten the risk of arthritis development.

- **Infections:** Certain infections can trigger types of arthritis, such as reactive arthritis.

Tips to Manage and Prevent Arthritis

Effective strategies to manage arthritis symptoms and reduce the risk of developing the condition include:

- **Stay Active:** Engage in regular exercise to strengthen muscles around joints, improve flexibility, and alleviate pain. Low-impact activities like walking, swimming, or yoga are gentle on the joints.

- **Protect Your Joints:** Avoid activities that place repetitive stress on joints. Use ergonomic tools and modify tasks to minimize joint strain. Utilize assistive devices such as splints, braces, or canes to support and safeguard joints during daily activities.

- **Use Hot and Cold Therapy:** Applying heat or cold packs to affected joints can help relieve pain and reduce inflammation.

- **Practice Physical Therapy:** Work with a physical therapist to develop a personalized exercise program and learn techniques to enhance joint function and mobility.

Importance of Regular Healthcare Checkups

Regular healthcare checkups are indispensable as we age, serving as a proactive approach to maintaining our health. Much like scheduling regular maintenance for a car to prevent breakdowns, these checkups are designed to catch potential health issues early, before they escalate into more serious problems. Our bodies undergo various changes with age, from shifts in metabolism to changes in organ function, making regular monitoring and early intervention essential components of staying healthy.

The primary benefit of regular checkups lies in their ability to detect health issues before symptoms appear. Conditions such as high blood pressure, diabetes, and high cholesterol often develop silently, posing significant risks like heart disease or stroke if left unchecked. By monitoring vital signs, blood tests, and other diagnostic measures during checkups, healthcare providers can identify abnormalities and initiate timely treatments or lifestyle interventions. This proactive approach not only enhances longevity but also improves overall quality of life by reducing the impact of chronic conditions.

Moreover, regular checkups offer personalized guidance tailored to individual health needs. Healthcare providers can offer advice on nutrition to support optimal health, recommend suitable exercise routines to maintain mobility and strength, and provide strategies for managing stress effectively. For those managing chronic conditions or taking medications, checkups ensure that treatments are adjusted as needed to achieve optimal health outcomes while minimizing side effects.

Preparing for a checkup involves more than just showing up; it is about actively engaging in your health management. By compiling questions and concerns beforehand, patients can make the most of their time with healthcare providers, ensuring that discussions are focused and productive. This collaborative approach empowers individuals to take charge of their health journey, fostering a partnership between patient and provider aimed at achieving and maintaining optimal health as we navigate the path of healthy aging.

As we approach the end of our journey, the next chapter will delve into practical tips for embracing healthy aging, summarizing all that we have learned so far.

Final Thoughts:

Embracing a Life of Healthy Aging

Everyone experiences aging, which can sometimes seem daunting. Concerns about wrinkles, fitness levels, and health can lead some to try various methods, such as costly beauty treatments or anti-aging products. However, with the insights gained from this book, you understand that aging, whether swift or gradual, can be a beautiful and manageable journey through proper education and positive lifestyle habits.

Thinking of aging as leveling up in a video game provides an interesting perspective. Each level presents unique challenges and rewards, much like aging does in real life. The key to healthy aging begins with maintaining a balanced diet that is abundant in essential nutrients. This involves consuming plenty of fruits, vegetables, whole grains, and lean proteins. These foods are rich in vitamins, minerals, and antioxidants that support overall bodily functions. Specifically, fruits and vegetables play a crucial role in combating oxidative stress caused by free radicals, which are associated with aging and various diseases.

Staying hydrated is crucial for overall health. Water plays a vital role in digestion, maintains skin hydration, and supports cognitive function, keeping your brain alert and sharp. Conversely, reducing the intake of processed foods, sugars, and unhealthy fats is advisable, as they can contribute to weight gain, heart problems, and diabetes, and may even promote cancerous cell growth.

Remaining physically active is essential for healthy aging. Regular exercise offers numerous benefits, including improved cardiovascular health, increased muscle strength, enhanced flexibility, and a boosted mood. Aerobic exercises such as walking, swimming, or biking are excellent for maintaining heart and lung health. Strength training exercises help preserve muscle mass and bone density, crucial for mobility and fracture prevention. Incorporating flexibility exercises like yoga or stretching can improve the range of motion and reduce the risk of injuries associated with stiffness.

Exercise not only benefits physical health but also has an impact on mental well-being. When you exercise, your body releases endorphins, often referred to as "feel-good" hormones, which can alleviate symptoms of depression and anxiety, promoting a positive mood. Moreover, physical activity enhances brain function by increasing blood flow and stimulating the growth of new brain cells, which can improve cognitive abilities.

Maintaining mental acuity is crucial for healthy aging. Engaging in activities like reading, solving puzzles, and learning new skills keeps your mind active and helps delay cognitive decline. These activities are beneficial for enhancing memory, attention span, and problem-solving abilities, ensuring that your brain remains sharp and resilient as you age. Incorporating these practices into your daily routine supports overall mental health and contributes to a fulfilling and vibrant life.

As you age, managing stress becomes crucial for maintaining overall health and well-being. Chronic stress can contribute to serious health conditions such as high blood pressure, heart disease, and mental health issues. Adopting stress management techniques like meditation, deep breathing exercises, and engaging in hobbies can effectively reduce stress levels, promote relaxation, and improve your overall mood.

Equally important for emotional and mental health is maintaining strong social connections. Human beings thrive on social interaction and staying connected with family, friends, and the community helps prevent feelings of loneliness and depression that are common among older adults. Interacting with others in a respectful and friendly manner not only provides emotional support but also fosters a sense of belonging and fulfillment.

Engaging in social activities, volunteering, or joining clubs can significantly enrich your life. These activities not only connect you with others but also stimulate your mind, enhance life satisfaction, and provide opportunities to contribute positively to your community. Giving back through volunteer work or social engagements can be incredibly rewarding, offering a sense of purpose and fulfillment as you navigate the aging process.

Preventive healthcare plays a crucial role in the early detection and management of health issues. By scheduling regular checkups, screenings, and vaccinations, individuals can identify conditions such as high blood pressure, diabetes, and cancer in their early stages, when treatment is most effective. Taking a proactive approach to health, including managing chronic illnesses through regular medical care, can prevent complications and enhance overall quality of life.

In addition to medical care, lifestyle choices are key factors in maintaining health and preventing chronic diseases. Maintaining a healthy weight, avoiding smoking, and limiting alcohol intake are important steps that can significantly reduce the risk of developing health problems. These lifestyle habits, combined with consistent medical checkups and preventive measures, contribute to keeping individuals healthy, active, and enjoying a high quality of life.

Adequate sleep is essential for optimal health and cognitive function. During sleep, the body undergoes crucial repair processes and consolidates memories. It plays a vital role in regulating mood and enhancing the immune system. Conversely, insufficient sleep can contribute to the development of serious health conditions such as heart disease, diabetes, obesity, and cognitive decline.

Establishing a consistent sleep routine and creating a restful sleep environment are key strategies to improve sleep quality. Going to bed at the same time each night helps regulate the body's internal clock, promoting better sleep patterns. Limiting screen time before bed reduces exposure to blue light, which can interfere with melatonin production and disrupt sleep. Additionally, ensuring your bedroom is comfortable—cool, quiet, and dark—promotes an environment conducive to restful sleep. By cultivating good sleep habits, you can wake up feeling refreshed and prepared to tackle the day ahead, supporting overall well-being and productivity.

Taking part in activities that bring you joy and fulfillment is integral to healthy aging and overall well-being. Finding meaning and purpose in life can significantly enhance your quality of life as you age. Engaging in hobbies, pursuing passions, and setting new goals are pathways to experiencing happiness and fulfillment.

Whether it is immersing yourself in a long-cherished hobby, exploring new interests, or contributing to your community, these activities enrich your life in profound ways. They provide opportunities for personal growth, creativity, and self-expression, which are vital for emotional well-being and maintaining a positive outlook.

Staying involved in activities you love not only boosts your mood but also fosters a sense of accomplishment and satisfaction. It keeps your mind active and engaged, promoting cognitive health and resilience. Embracing new experiences adds excitement and variety to your daily life, making each day meaningful and rewarding.

By prioritizing activities that bring you joy and fulfillment, you cultivate a fulfilling and vibrant life, fostering happiness and well-being as you navigate the journey of healthy aging.

In summary, healthy aging entails adopting a holistic approach to well-being and embracing life with vitality and optimism. One of its most significant rewards is the preservation of independence. By prioritizing healthy aging practices, you can elevate your quality of life, remain confidently self-reliant, and embark on a vibrant, fulfilling journey through the years.

The habits you cultivate today profoundly shape your future well-being. By adopting a healthy lifestyle now, you are investing in a future where you can continue to enjoy life's pleasures without the typical limitations associated with aging. Take small steps each day toward a healthier lifestyle and celebrate every milestone along the way. Your future self will deeply appreciate the commitment and care you show today.

Aging brings numerous positives. With each passing year, you accumulate more knowledge and experience, which empowers you to navigate life's challenges with greater wisdom and grace. Embrace the confidence that stems from your experiences and use it to enrich not only your own life but also the lives of those around you. Surround yourself with positive and supportive individuals who uplift and inspire you.

Embracing the aging process is about cherishing the journey of your life. Appreciate the wisdom and resilience that come with age, focusing on what you can control while maintaining a positive outlook. Stay curious, nurture meaningful relationships, and find purpose in your experiences to gracefully and joyfully navigate the passage of time.

Remember, aging is not just about growing older; it is about growing wiser, stronger, and more resilient with each passing day.

References

Adaes, S. (2024, February 20). *Mitochondria: 10 ways to boost the powerhouse of your cells.* Dr. Axe. https://draxe.com/health/mitochondria/

Bryan, S., Afful, J., Carroll, M., Te-Ching, C., Orlando, D., Fink, S., & Fryar, C. (2021, June 14). *NHSR 158. National health and nutrition examination survey 2017–march 2020 pre-pandemic data files.* Centers for Disease Control and Prevention. https://stacks.cdc.gov/view/cdc/106273

De Lorenzo, A., Gratteri, S., Gualtieri, P., Cammarano, A., Bertucci, P., & Di Renzo, L. (2019). Why primary obesity is a disease? *Journal of Translational Medicine, 17*(1). https://doi.org/10.1186/s12967-019-1919-y

Fallis, J. (2024, February 20). *25 powerful ways to boost the mitochondria in your brain.* Optimal Living Dynamics. https://www.optimallivingdynamics.com/blog/how-to-support-your-mitochondria-for-better-brain-health-mental-boost-increase-optimize-restore-repair-function-depression-fatigue-energy-foods-supplements-naturally-biogenesis

Flynn, H. (2023, December 2). *Longevity: Healthier diet at age 40 could add 8 years to your life.* Medical News Today. https://www.medicalnewstoday.com/articles/switching-to-a-healthier-diet-linked-to-improved-longevity#How-healthy-diets-impact-longevity

George, G. A., & Heaton, F. W. (1975). Changes in cellular composition during magnesium deficiency. *Biochemical Journal, 152*(3), 609–615. http://www.ncbi.nlm.nih.gov/pmc/articles/PMC1172515/

Luders, E., Toga, A. W., Lepore, N., & Gaser, C. (2009). The underlying anatomical correlates of long-term meditation: Larger hippocampal and frontal volumes of gray matter. *NeuroImage*, *45*(3), 672–678. https://www.ncbi.nlm.nih.gov/pmc/articles/PMC3184843/

Miller, A. (2021, September 25). *What is methylation and why should you care about it*. Thorne. https://www.thorne.com/take-5-daily/article/what-is-methylation-and-why-should-you-care-about-it

Pan American Health Organization. (n.d.). *Healthy aging*. PAHO. https://www.paho.org/en/healthy-aging

Protect your brain from stress. (2018, August 1). Harvard Health. https://www.health.harvard.edu/mind-and-mood/protect-your-brain-from-stress#:~:text=Stress%20management%20may%20reduce%20health

Silberman, S. (2022, April 21). *The national council on aging*. NCOA. https://www.ncoa.org/article/the-inequities-in-the-cost-of-chronic-disease-why-it-matters-for-older-adults

Ware, M. (2020, January 6). *Magnesium: Health benefits, deficiency, sources, and risks*. Medical News Today. https://www.medicalnewstoday.com/articles/286839

Yau, S., Gil-Mohapel, J., Christie, B. R., & So, K. (2014). Physical exercise-induced adult neurogenesis: A good strategy to prevent cognitive decline in neurodegenerative diseases? *BioMed Research International*, *2014*, 1–20. https://doi.org/10.1155/2014/403120

Image References

Any Lane. (2020, November 21). *Delicious multicolored apples and oranges with mandarins located in red bowl* [Image]. Pexels. https://www.pexels.com/photo/delicious-multicolored-apples-and-oranges-with-mandarins-located-in-red-bowl-5945899/

Ketut Subiyanto. (2020, July 12). *Man and Woman Exercise Together* [Image]. Pexels. https://www.pexels.com/photo/man-and-woman-exercise-together-4853077/

Marcus Aurelius. (2021, February 11). *Woman Doing Warrior Pose* [Image]. Pexels. https://www.pexels.com/photo/woman-doing-warrior-pose-6787161/

Yan Krukau. (2021, July 4). *Active Kids Doing Bending Exercise* [Image]. Pexels. https://www.pexels.com/photo/active-kids-doing-bending-exercise-8613305/